Natural Remedies to

Sustain Me

In Life with

Barbara O'Neill's

Guidance book

A Complete Guide to Natural Remedies and Herbal Treatments for Holistic Health

Dr. E. Neil

Table of Contents

- Introduction: The Path to Lasting Wellness 1

The Limitations of Quick Fixes and Fad Diets...1

Embracing a Holistic Approach to Health 3

PART ONE: UNDERSTANDING THE PRINCIPLES OF SUSTAIN ME...................................7

Chapter 1: S - Sustenance 8

The Role of Nutrition in Overall Health...8

Building a Balanced Diet: Foods to Embrace and Avoid...11

The Impact of Processed Foods and How to Transition to Whole Foods 16

Chapter 2: U – Unwind 21

The Importance of Stress Management for Well-Being...21

Techniques for Relaxation and Mental Clarity 25

Incorporating Mindfulness and Meditation into Daily Life 29

Chapter 3: S – Sleep 35

Understanding the Science of Sleep 35

Creating Healthy Sleep Habits for Restorative Rest...39

The Connection Between Sleep and Immune Function...44

Chapter 4: T - Toxin Elimination 48

   Detoxifying Your Body Naturally..48

   The Role of Liver and Kidney Health in Detoxification..52

   Using Herbs and Supplements to Support Detoxification 55

Chapter 5: A – Activity...59

   The Benefits of Regular Physical Exercise..59

   Choosing the Right Type of Exercise for Your Body...62

   Integrating Movement into a Busy Lifestyle..65

Chapter 6: I - Immune Support...68

   Strengthening Your Immune System Naturally 68

   The Role of Nutrition, Sleep, and Stress Management in Immunity 72

   Herbal Remedies and Supplements for Immune Health......................................74

Chapter 7: N - Nourish..79

   Understanding the Concept of Nourishment Beyond Food 79

   The Role of Emotional and Spiritual Health in Physical Well-Being..................82

   Building Resilience Through Positive Relationships and Community..................84

Chapter 8: M – Mindset..89

    The Power of Positive Thinking in Healing...89

    Cultivating a Growth Mindset for Lifelong Wellness 93

    Strategies for Overcoming Negative Thoughts and Emotions...........98

Chapter 9: E – Empower..103

    Taking Control of Your Health Journey...103

    Building Confidence in Your Ability to Heal.......................................107

    Creating a Sustainable Wellness Plan...112

PART TWO: PRACTICAL APPLICATIONS 117

Chapter 10: Integrating the SUSTAIN ME Principles 118

    Creating a Personalized Wellness Plan 118

    Tracking Progress and Making Adjustments.....................................123

    Overcoming Common Challenges...127

Chapter 11: Herbal Remedies and Natural Solutions 132

    An Introduction to Herbal Medicine..132

    Key Herbs for Common Ailments...135

How to Prepare and Use Herbal Remedies Safely 139

Chapter 12: Nutrition and Meal Planning 143

Developing a Balanced Meal Plan 143

Recipes for Health and Vitality 148

Adapting Your Diet for Different Life Stages and Needs...154

PART THREE: ADVANCED TOPICS 158

Chapter 13: Functional Medicine and Holistic Health 159

The Role of Functional Medicine in Modern Healthcare 159

Integrating Functional Medicine Principles into Your Life 162

Case Studies and Success Stories 167

Chapter 14: Preventing and Reversing Chronic Illness 172

Understanding the Root Causes of Chronic Diseases..172

Strategies for Prevention and Reversal 174

The Role of Lifestyle Medicine in Chronic Disease Management...............................179

Chapter 15: Living a Life of Vibrant Health 183

Cultivating Long-Term Wellness Habits..183

Finding Joy and Purpose in Healthful Living 186

Inspiring Stories of Transformation...189

Conclusion: Your Journey to Optimal Health...193

Reflecting on the SUSTAIN ME Principles..193

Continuing Your Wellness Journey 196

Encouraging Others to Embrace a Holistic Lifestyle 199

Introduction: The Path to Lasting Wellness

The Limitations of Quick Fixes and Fad Diets

In today's fast-paced world, the allure of quick fixes and fad diets is stronger than ever. Promises of rapid weight loss, detoxification, or instant energy boost are tempting, especially for those seeking immediate results. However, the reality of these trendy solutions often falls short of their promises, leading to frustration, disappointment, and even negative health consequences.

The Illusion of Immediate Results

Quick fixes and fad diets are often marketed with bold claims of fast results, but these outcomes are typically short-lived. Many of these diets work by severely restricting calories, cutting out entire food groups, or promoting the excessive consumption of certain "Super-foods." While these methods may lead to initial weight loss or other noticeable changes, they are rarely sustainable. Once the diet is abandoned, which often happens due to its restrictive nature, the weight is usually regained, sometimes even more than before.

This cycle of rapid weight loss followed by equally rapid weight gain, often referred to as "yo-yo dieting," can have serious repercussions on one's metabolism. The body, perceiving the restriction as a threat, may slow down its metabolic rate to conserve energy, making it harder to lose weight in the future and easier to gain it back.

Nutritional Imbalance and Health Risks

Fad diets often involve extreme dietary measures that can lead to nutritional imbalances. For example, diets that eliminate entire food groups, such as carbohydrates or fats, deprive the body of essential nutrients that are crucial for overall health. Carbohydrates, particularly complex ones, are vital for energy production and brain function, while healthy fats are necessary for hormone production, cell structure, and nutrient absorption.

Moreover, the focus on a single nutrient or food group can result in overconsumption, leading to other health issues. For instance, high-protein diets might stress the kidneys, while low-carb diets could lead to fatigue, digestive issues, and a lack of dietary fiber, essential for gut health.

In the pursuit of quick results, many people neglect the importance of a balanced, varied diet that provides all the necessary nutrients in appropriate amounts. This imbalance can weaken the immune system, decrease energy levels, and even increase the risk of chronic diseases such as heart disease, diabetes, and osteoporosis.

The Psychological Toll

Beyond the physical health risks, quick fixes and fad diets can take a significant toll on mental and emotional well-being. The restrictive nature of these diets can lead to feelings of deprivation, frustration, and guilt, especially when "cheating" or deviating from the plan. This can create an unhealthy relationship with food, where eating becomes associated with stress, anxiety, and shame.

Furthermore, the constant focus on dieting and body image can foster a negative self-image and contribute to the development of eating disorders. The obsession with achieving a certain body type, often perpetuated by social media and celebrity culture, can lead to an endless cycle of dieting, dissatisfaction, and emotional distress.

Lack of Long-Term Sustainability

One of the most significant limitations of quick fixes and fad diets is their lack of long-term sustainability. These diets often require drastic changes that are difficult to maintain over time, leading to a high rate of failure. The restrictive rules and rigid structure can be challenging to integrate into daily life, especially when it comes to social events, travel, and family meals.

In contrast, a sustainable approach to health and wellness involves gradual, realistic changes that can be maintained over the long term. It focuses on creating a balanced diet, regular physical activity, stress management, and a positive mindset. This holistic approach not only supports weight management but also enhances overall well-being, reduces the risk of chronic diseases, and promotes a healthier, more fulfilling life.

The Importance of a Holistic Approach

The limitations of quick fixes and fad diets underscore the need for a holistic approach to health and wellness. Rather than chasing after the latest diet trend, it is essential to focus on creating a balanced, nutrient-rich diet that supports the body's needs. This approach involves listening to the body's signals, understanding individual nutritional requirements, and making informed choices that promote long-term health.

A holistic approach also emphasizes the importance of regular physical activity, adequate sleep, stress management, and emotional well-being. It recognizes that true health is not just about achieving a certain weight or body shape but about feeling good, having energy, and living a balanced, fulfilling life.

In conclusion, while quick fixes and fad diets may offer the promise of immediate results, they often fail to deliver sustainable, long-term health benefits. By embracing a holistic approach to wellness, individuals can achieve lasting results that enhance their quality of life and support overall well-being.

Embracing a Holistic Approach to Health

In a world where modern medicine often focuses on treating symptoms rather than addressing the root causes of health issues, embracing a holistic approach to health offers a pathway to true well-being. This approach considers the whole person—body, mind, and spirit—and emphasizes the interconnectedness of various aspects of life. By integrating physical health, mental clarity, emotional balance, and spiritual fulfillment, a holistic approach aims to achieve lasting wellness.

The Foundation of Holistic Health

Holistic health is built on the understanding that the body is a complex, interdependent system where every part influences the others. Rather than isolating a problem or treating a single symptom, holistic health practitioners seek to understand the underlying causes of health issues and how they relate to the overall well-being of the individual.

This approach is rooted in the belief that optimal health is achieved through balance. This balance encompasses various facets of life, including nutrition, exercise, sleep, stress management, emotional well-being, and spiritual practices. Each element plays a crucial role in maintaining health, and neglecting one aspect can disrupt the harmony of the whole.

Nutrition as a Cornerstone

In holistic health, nutrition is seen as one of the primary pillars of well-being. The food we consume directly impacts our physical health, energy levels, and mental clarity. A holistic approach to nutrition focuses on eating whole, unprocessed foods that are rich in nutrients and free from harmful additives. This means prioritizing fresh fruits and vegetables, whole grains, healthy fats, and lean proteins while minimizing processed foods, refined sugars, and artificial ingredients.

But holistic nutrition goes beyond just what we eat; it also considers how we eat. Mindful eating—paying attention to hunger cues, eating slowly, and savoring each bite—helps to improve digestion, foster a healthy relationship with food, and prevent overeating. Additionally, understanding the body's unique nutritional needs and adjusting the diet accordingly can help address specific health concerns and enhance overall well-being.

The Importance of Physical Activity

Regular physical activity is another essential component of holistic health. Exercise is not only vital for maintaining a healthy weight, but it also supports cardiovascular health, boosts the immune system, enhances mood, and promotes better sleep. A holistic approach to exercise encourages finding activities that are enjoyable and sustainable, whether it's yoga, walking, swimming, or strength training.

The key is to view exercise not as a chore but as a form of self-care that contributes to overall health and happiness. Incorporating movement into daily routines, whether through structured workouts or simply staying active throughout the day, is fundamental to maintaining physical and mental well-being.

Managing Stress and Emotional Health

Stress is an unavoidable part of life, but chronic stress can have detrimental effects on health. A holistic approach recognizes the importance of managing stress to prevent it from leading to more serious health issues, such as anxiety, depression, or chronic illness. Techniques like deep breathing, meditation, mindfulness, and yoga are often recommended to help calm the mind and reduce stress levels.

Emotional health is equally important in a holistic approach. Emotions are deeply intertwined with physical health, and unresolved emotional issues can manifest as physical symptoms. Holistic health encourages practices like journaling, therapy, or simply talking with a trusted friend to process emotions and maintain emotional balance.

Sleep: The Body's Natural Healer

Sleep is a critical, yet often overlooked, component of holistic health. Quality sleep allows the body to repair and regenerate, supports cognitive function, and regulates mood. A holistic approach emphasizes the importance of creating healthy sleep habits, such as maintaining a consistent sleep schedule, creating a restful environment, and avoiding stimulants before bedtime.

Recognizing the connection between sleep and overall health, holistic practices often incorporate techniques to improve sleep quality, such as relaxation exercises, herbal remedies, and adjusting diet and lifestyle factors that may be disrupting sleep.

Spiritual Well-being and Purpose

Spiritual health is a personal and often misunderstood aspect of holistic well-being. It doesn't necessarily refer to religion but rather to a sense of purpose, connection, and inner peace. For some, this might mean connecting with nature, practicing gratitude, engaging in community service, or simply spending time in reflection or meditation.

Embracing spiritual practices can provide a sense of fulfillment, reduce stress, and offer a deeper understanding of one's place in the world. It is about nurturing the soul and finding meaning in life's experiences.

Integrating Holistic Health into Daily Life

Adopting a holistic approach to health is not about making radical changes overnight but about gradually integrating healthy habits into daily life. It requires self-awareness, a willingness to listen to the body's signals, and a commitment to making choices that support overall well-being.

Start by making small, manageable changes, such as incorporating more whole foods into your diet, finding time for regular physical activity, or setting aside moments for relaxation and reflection. Over time, these small changes can lead to significant improvements in health and quality of life.

In conclusion, embracing a holistic approach to health is about nurturing the entire self—physically, mentally, emotionally, and spiritually. By focusing on the whole person and recognizing the interconnectedness of all aspects of life, holistic health offers a path to true and lasting wellness, one that empowers individuals to live balanced, fulfilling lives.

PART ONE: UNDERSTANDING THE PRINCIPLES OF SUSTAIN ME

Chapter 1: S - Sustenance

The Role of Nutrition in Overall Health

Nutrition plays a fundamental role in maintaining and enhancing overall health. It is the foundation upon which our physical, mental, and emotional well-being is built. Proper nutrition provides the body with essential nutrients, including vitamins, minerals, proteins, fats, and carbohydrates, which are necessary for growth, energy, and the functioning of vital organs. Understanding the importance of nutrition and making informed dietary choices can lead to a longer, healthier life and prevent the onset of chronic diseases.

Nutrients: The Building Blocks of Health

Our bodies rely on a variety of nutrients to perform essential functions. These nutrients can be broadly categorized into macronutrients and micronutrients:

- **Macronutrients** include carbohydrates, proteins, and fats. They provide energy, support growth and repair, and regulate bodily processes.

    o **Carbohydrates** are the body's primary source of energy, fueling daily activities and brain function.

    o **Proteins** are crucial for building and repairing tissues, producing enzymes and hormones, and supporting immune function.

    o **Fats** are vital for energy storage, protecting organs, insulating the body, and aiding in the absorption of fat-soluble vitamins.

- **Micronutrients** include vitamins and minerals that are needed in smaller amounts but are equally essential for health.

    o **Vitamins** like A, C, D, E, and B-complex support immune function, skin health, bone strength, and energy production.

o **Minerals** such as calcium, magnesium, potassium, and iron are necessary for bone health, muscle function, fluid balance, and oxygen transport.

Each nutrient has a specific role in maintaining the body's complex systems. A deficiency in any of these nutrients can lead to health problems, while a balanced intake ensures that the body functions optimally.

Nutrition and Chronic Disease Prevention

A well-balanced diet is one of the most effective tools for preventing chronic diseases, such as heart disease, diabetes, obesity, and certain cancers. Poor nutrition, characterized by diets high in processed foods, added sugars, unhealthy fats, and low in fruits, vegetables, and whole grains, is a significant risk factor for these conditions.

- **Heart Health:** A diet rich in fruits, vegetables, whole grains, lean proteins, and healthy fats (like omega-3 fatty acids from fish and nuts) can help maintain healthy cholesterol levels, reduce blood pressure, and lower the risk of heart disease.

- **Diabetes Management:** For those with or at risk of diabetes, managing carbohydrate intake, choosing whole grains over refined grains, and including fiber-rich foods can help regulate blood sugar levels and improve insulin sensitivity.

- **Weight Management:** Balanced nutrition, when combined with regular physical activity, helps maintain a healthy weight, which is crucial for reducing the risk of obesity-related conditions like hypertension, type 2 diabetes, and joint problems.

- **Cancer Prevention:** Certain nutrients and dietary patterns have been linked to a reduced risk of cancer. For example, diets high in fruits and vegetables provide antioxidants that protect cells from damage, while limiting processed meats and reducing alcohol intake can lower cancer risk.

The Gut-Brain Connection

Nutrition also plays a crucial role in mental health, largely due to the gut-brain connection. The gut, often referred to as the "second brain," houses trillions of bacteria that influence mood, cognitive function, and overall mental well-being. A diet rich in fiber, prebiotics, and probiotics supports a healthy gut microbiome, which in turn can reduce inflammation and improve mood disorders like anxiety and depression.

- **Mood and Cognitive Function:** Nutrients like omega-3 fatty acids, found in fatty fish, and antioxidants from fruits and vegetables have been shown to support brain health, enhance cognitive function, and reduce the risk of neurodegenerative diseases like Alzheimer's.

- **Stress and Anxiety:** Foods high in magnesium, such as leafy greens, nuts, and seeds, can help reduce stress and anxiety. Similarly, maintaining stable blood sugar levels through balanced meals can prevent mood swings and irritability.

Immune Function and Healing

Nutrition is integral to a strong immune system and the body's ability to heal and recover from illness or injury. Vitamins and minerals like vitamin C, vitamin D, zinc, and selenium play key roles in immune function, helping to fend off infections and support the body's natural healing processes.

- **Immune Support:** Consuming a variety of colorful fruits and vegetables ensures a robust intake of antioxidants and phytonutrients, which protect against oxidative stress and bolster the immune system.

- **Healing and Recovery:** Protein is vital for tissue repair and recovery after injury or surgery. Additionally, anti-inflammatory foods such as leafy greens, berries, and fatty fish can help reduce inflammation and speed up the healing process.

Personalized Nutrition: One Size Does Not Fit All

It's important to recognize that nutrition is not a one-size-fits-all concept. Individual nutritional needs can vary based on age, gender, activity level, health status, and genetic factors. Personalized nutrition takes into account these differences, allowing for tailored dietary recommendations that address specific health goals and conditions.

For instance, an athlete may require more protein and carbohydrates to fuel performance and recovery, while someone with a sedentary lifestyle may need fewer calories and more nutrient-dense foods to maintain a healthy weight. Similarly, those with food intolerances or allergies need to modify their diets to avoid triggers while still meeting their nutritional needs.

Sustainable Eating: The Bigger Picture

In addition to personal health, nutrition choices also have broader implications for environmental sustainability and social well-being. Choosing locally sourced, organic, and plant-based foods can reduce one's carbon footprint and support ethical food production practices. Sustainable eating encourages a mindful approach to food, considering not only the impact on personal health but also the health of the planet.

Nutrition is a powerful tool for maintaining health, preventing disease, and enhancing overall well-being. By making informed dietary choices and understanding the vital role of nutrients in the body, individuals can take control of their health and pave the way for a vibrant, fulfilling life. Embracing a balanced, whole-foods-based diet, tailored to individual needs and preferences, is the cornerstone of lasting wellness.

Building a Balanced Diet: Foods to Embrace and Avoid

A balanced diet is the cornerstone of good health, providing the essential nutrients our bodies need to function optimally. It is about more than just counting calories; it's about making mindful choices that promote well-being, prevent disease, and support long-term health. Understanding which foods to embrace and which to avoid is crucial in crafting a diet that meets your nutritional needs and supports overall wellness.

The Foundation of a Balanced Diet

A balanced diet includes a variety of foods from different food groups, ensuring that you get the necessary macronutrients (carbohydrates, proteins, and fats) and micronutrients (vitamins and minerals). The key is to focus on whole, minimally processed foods that provide high nutritional value while avoiding those that can negatively impact health.

Foods to Embrace

1. **Fruits and Vegetables:**

   o **Benefits:** Rich in vitamins, minerals, fiber, and antioxidants, fruits and vegetables are vital for immune function, digestion, and reducing the risk of chronic diseases.

   o **Variety:** Aim for a colorful array, including leafy greens (like spinach and kale), cruciferous vegetables (like broccoli and cauliflower), and fruits high in vitamin C (like oranges and berries).

   o **Serving Recommendation:** At least five servings of fruits and vegetables per day, with an emphasis on vegetables for their lower sugar content.

2. **Whole Grains:**

   o **Benefits:** Whole grains like brown rice, quinoa, oats, and whole wheat provide fiber, B vitamins, and essential minerals. They support digestion, regulate blood sugar, and promote heart health.

   o **Serving Recommendation:** Replace refined grains with whole grains in your diet, aiming for at least three servings per day.

3. **Lean Proteins:**

   o **Benefits:** Proteins are essential for muscle repair, enzyme production, and immune function. Lean sources such as poultry, fish, beans, legumes, and tofu provide high-quality protein without excess saturated fat.

   o **Fish:** Fatty fish like salmon, mackerel, and sardines are excellent sources of omega-3 fatty acids, which support heart and brain health.

   o **Serving Recommendation:** Include a variety of protein sources in your diet, with an emphasis on plant-based proteins and fatty fish.

4. **Healthy Fats:**

   o **Benefits:** Healthy fats, including those from nuts, seeds, avocados, and olive oil, are essential for brain health, hormone production, and cellular function.

- **Omega-3s:** Omega-3 fatty acids, found in flaxseeds, walnuts, and fish, are particularly beneficial for reducing inflammation and supporting cardiovascular health.

- **Serving Recommendation:** Incorporate healthy fats into your daily diet, focusing on unsaturated fats while limiting saturated and trans fats.

5. **Dairy or Dairy Alternatives:**

- **Benefits:** Dairy products like yogurt, cheese, and milk provide calcium, vitamin D, and protein. For those who are lactose intolerant or prefer plant-based options, fortified alternatives like almond milk or soy yogurt can offer similar benefits.

- **Serving Recommendation:** Include moderate amounts of dairy or fortified alternatives to support bone health.

6. **Hydration:**

- **Importance:** Proper hydration is crucial for digestion, circulation, temperature regulation, and overall cellular function.

- **Water:** Water should be your primary beverage, but herbal teas and water-rich fruits and vegetables also contribute to hydration.

- **Recommendation:** Aim to drink at least 8 glasses (about 2 liters) of water per day, adjusting for activity level and climate.

Foods to Avoid

1. **Processed Foods:**

- **Risks:** Processed foods often contain high levels of added sugars, unhealthy fats, sodium, and artificial additives. Regular consumption can lead to obesity, heart disease, and other chronic conditions.

- **Examples:** Packaged snacks, sugary cereals, processed meats, and fast food.

- **Recommendation:** Minimize processed food intake, focusing instead on whole, natural foods.

2. **Sugary Beverages and Snacks:**

o **Risks:** High sugar intake is linked to weight gain, type 2 diabetes, and dental problems. Sugary drinks like sodas, energy drinks, and sweetened teas are major contributors to excess calorie intake without nutritional benefit.

o **Examples:** Sodas, candies, pastries, and sweetened breakfast cereals.

o **Recommendation:** Replace sugary drinks with water, herbal teas, or diluted fruit juices. Choose whole fruits instead of sugary snacks.

3. **Refined Grains:**

o **Risks:** Refined grains, such as white bread, white rice, and pastries, have been stripped of their fiber and nutrients, leading to rapid spikes in blood sugar and increased risk of insulin resistance.

o **Examples:** White bread, white pasta, and most commercially baked goods.

o **Recommendation:** Opt for whole grains whenever possible and limit consumption of refined grains.

4. **Trans Fats and Saturated Fats:**

o **Risks:** Trans fats, often found in fried foods, baked goods, and margarine, increase the risk of heart disease by raising bad cholesterol (LDL) and lowering good cholesterol (HDL). Saturated fats, found in fatty cuts of meat, butter, and full-fat dairy, can also contribute to cardiovascular disease when consumed in excess.

o **Examples:** Fried fast food, margarine, and commercially prepared baked goods.

o **Recommendation:** Avoid trans fats entirely and limit saturated fats, choosing healthier fat sources like olive oil and nuts.

5. **Excessive Sodium:**

- **Risks:** High sodium intake is linked to hypertension, heart disease, and stroke. Processed and packaged foods are often high in sodium, making it easy to exceed the recommended daily intake.

- **Examples:** Processed meats, canned soups, salty snacks, and restaurant meals.

- **Recommendation:** Limit sodium intake by choosing fresh, unprocessed foods and using herbs and spices to flavor meals instead of salt.

6. **Alcohol in Excess:**

- **Risks:** While moderate alcohol consumption can be part of a balanced diet for some, excessive intake is associated with liver disease, certain cancers, and mental health disorders.

- **Recommendation:** If you choose to drink, do so in moderation—up to one drink per day for women and two for men.

Creating a Balanced Plate

Building a balanced diet involves not only selecting the right foods but also understanding portion control and variety. A balanced plate typically includes:

- **Half the plate filled with vegetables and fruits:** This ensures a high intake of fiber, vitamins, and minerals.

- **One-quarter of the plate with lean proteins:** To support muscle repair and overall bodily function.

- **One-quarter of the plate with whole grains:** For sustained energy and digestive health.

- **A small amount of healthy fats:** Such as a drizzle of olive oil or a handful of nuts.

Practical Tips for Building a Balanced Diet

- **Meal Planning:** Plan meals ahead of time to ensure a balanced diet and reduce the temptation of unhealthy options.

- **Mindful Eating:** Pay attention to hunger and fullness cues, and enjoy your food without distractions.

- **Cooking at Home:** Prepare meals at home to have more control over ingredients and portion sizes.

- **Reading Labels:** Learn to read food labels to make informed choices, paying attention to ingredients, serving sizes, and nutritional content.

- **Gradual Changes:** If transitioning to a healthier diet, make gradual changes to avoid feeling overwhelmed.

Building a balanced diet is about making choices that nourish the body, support health, and prevent disease. By embracing whole, nutrient-rich foods and avoiding processed, high-sugar, and high-fat options, you can create a sustainable and enjoyable eating pattern that promotes long-term wellness. Remember, balance and variety are key, ensuring that your diet provides all the nutrients your body needs to thrive.

The Impact of Processed Foods and How to Transition to Whole Foods

Processed foods have become a staple in modern diets, offering convenience and longer shelf life. However, these foods often come with hidden costs to our health, contributing to a range of chronic diseases and undermining our well-being. Understanding the impact of processed foods and learning how to transition to whole foods is crucial for those seeking to improve their health and vitality.

The Impact of Processed Foods on Health

Processed foods are typically defined as foods that have been altered from their natural state through methods such as canning, freezing, refrigeration, dehydration, and aseptic processing. While some processing is necessary to make foods safe or more convenient to eat, many processed foods are laden with unhealthy ingredients that can have detrimental effects on health.

Nutritional Depletion

- **Loss of Nutrients:** Processing often strips foods of essential nutrients, including fiber, vitamins, and minerals. For example, refining grains removes the bran and germ, which contain the bulk of the fiber and nutrients.

- **Added Sugars and Unhealthy Fats:** To improve flavor and texture, processed foods often contain added sugars, unhealthy fats, and salt. These additives contribute to weight gain, heart disease, and diabetes.

- **Artificial Additives:** Many processed foods contain artificial colors, flavors, and preservatives that have been linked to various health issues, including allergies and hyperactivity in children.

Metabolic Effects

- **Blood Sugar Spikes:** Processed foods, particularly those high in refined carbohydrates and sugars, can cause rapid spikes in blood sugar levels. This can lead to insulin resistance, a precursor to type 2 diabetes.

- **Increased Caloric Intake:** Processed foods are often energy-dense and low in satiety, meaning they provide a lot of calories without making you feel full. This can lead to overeating and obesity.

- **Impaired Gut Health:** The lack of fiber and the presence of artificial ingredients in processed foods can negatively affect gut health, leading to issues like constipation, inflammation, and an imbalance in gut bacteria.

Long-Term Health Risks

- **Chronic Diseases:** Diets high in processed foods have been linked to an increased risk of chronic diseases such as heart disease, stroke, diabetes, and certain types of cancer.

- **Inflammation:** Processed foods often contain trans fats, refined sugars, and artificial additives that contribute to chronic inflammation, a root cause of many diseases.

- **Mental Health:** Emerging research suggests a link between processed food consumption and mental health issues, including depression and anxiety, possibly due to nutrient deficiencies and inflammatory effects.

Transitioning to Whole Foods

Making the shift from processed foods to whole foods is a powerful step toward improving your health. Whole foods are minimally processed and remain as close to their natural state as possible, retaining their full nutritional value. Transitioning to a whole-foods diet involves making mindful choices, planning ahead, and gradually changing your eating habits.

Steps to Transition to Whole Foods

1. **Start with Small Changes:**

   o **Gradual Replacement:** Begin by replacing one processed food item with a whole food alternative. For example, swap sugary cereals for oatmeal or replace white bread with whole grain bread.

   o **Focus on One Meal:** Start by making one meal a day entirely from whole foods, such as a homemade salad for lunch or a stir-fry with fresh vegetables and lean protein for dinner.

2. **Plan Your Meals:**

   o **Meal Prep:** Prepare meals and snacks ahead of time to avoid the temptation of processed foods. Having healthy options readily available makes it easier to stick to a whole-foods diet.

   o **Grocery List:** Make a list before shopping, focusing on whole foods like fruits, vegetables, whole grains, nuts, seeds, and lean proteins. Avoid the processed food aisles as much as possible.

3. **Read Food Labels:**

   o **Ingredient Awareness:** When buying packaged foods, read the ingredient list carefully. Choose products with fewer ingredients and avoid those with added sugars, artificial additives, and unhealthy fats.

- **Avoiding Marketing Traps:** Be cautious of marketing terms like "natural" or "healthy," which can be misleading. Always check the nutritional information and ingredients to ensure you are making a wise choice.

4. **Cook at Home:**

- **Homemade Meals:** Cooking at home allows you to control the ingredients and avoid hidden additives found in restaurant and processed foods. Experiment with new recipes that emphasize whole foods.

- **Batch Cooking:** Prepare large portions of meals and freeze them for later use. This can save time and reduce reliance on processed convenience foods.

5. **Focus on Whole Grains:**

- **Switch to Whole Grains:** Replace refined grains with whole grains like brown rice, quinoa, and oats. These grains retain their fiber and nutrients, supporting better digestion and sustained energy.

- **Whole Grain Products:** Look for whole grain versions of bread, pasta, and cereals. Ensure that "whole grain" is listed as the first ingredient.

6. **Increase Fruit and Vegetable Intake:**

- **Incorporate More Produce:** Aim to fill half your plate with fruits and vegetables at each meal. This increases your intake of essential vitamins, minerals, and antioxidants.

- **Seasonal and Local:** Choose seasonal and locally grown produce when possible, as they are often fresher and more nutritious.

7. **Choose Healthy Fats:**

- **Healthy Fat Sources:** Replace unhealthy fats found in processed foods with healthy fats from avocados, nuts, seeds, and olive oil. These fats support heart health and brain function.

- **Limit Processed Oils:** Avoid processed oils like canola and soybean oil, which are often high in omega-6 fatty acids that can contribute to inflammation.

8. **Stay Hydrated:**

   o **Drink Water:** Replace sugary drinks and sodas with water, herbal teas, or infused water with fruits and herbs. Proper hydration is essential for digestion, energy levels, and overall health.

Overcoming Challenges

- **Time Constraints:** The perceived time commitment of preparing whole foods can be a barrier. Address this by meal planning, using time-saving kitchen tools, and preparing meals in batches.

- **Budget Concerns:** Whole foods can sometimes be more expensive than processed options. Shop seasonally, buy in bulk, and prioritize spending on nutrient-dense foods.

- **Cravings for Processed Foods:** Gradually reduce the consumption of processed foods to decrease cravings. Find healthier alternatives and focus on the positive benefits of your new diet.

Benefits of Whole Foods

Transitioning to whole foods offers numerous health benefits, including improved energy levels, better digestion, weight management, and a reduced risk of chronic diseases. Whole foods provide the body with the nutrients it needs to function optimally, support immune health, and promote overall well-being. Additionally, a whole-foods diet is often more satisfying and enjoyable, as it allows you to appreciate the natural flavors and textures of foods.

The impact of processed foods on health is significant, contributing to a range of health issues from obesity to chronic diseases. Transitioning to a whole-foods diet is a powerful way to reclaim your health, providing your body with the nutrients it needs to thrive. By making gradual changes, planning ahead, and focusing on the benefits of whole foods, you can create a sustainable and healthful eating pattern that supports long-term wellness.

Chapter 2: U – Unwind

The Importance of Stress Management for Well-Being

Stress is an inevitable part of life, but how we manage it plays a crucial role in our overall well-being. While some stress can be motivating and even beneficial, chronic stress has detrimental effects on both physical and mental health. Understanding the importance of stress management and implementing effective strategies can lead to a more balanced, healthy, and fulfilling life.

The Nature of Stress

Stress is the body's response to perceived threats or challenges. It triggers the release of hormones like cortisol and adrenaline, preparing the body for a "fight or flight" reaction. This response is useful in short bursts, helping us respond to immediate dangers. However, when stress becomes chronic, it can lead to various health problems.

Physical Effects of Stress

- **Immune System Suppression:** Chronic stress weakens the immune system, making the body more susceptible to infections and illnesses.

- **Cardiovascular Strain:** Prolonged stress increases the risk of hypertension, heart disease, and stroke due to constant elevated blood pressure and heart rate.

- **Digestive Issues:** Stress can disrupt digestion, leading to conditions such as irritable bowel syndrome (IBS), acid reflux, and other gastrointestinal problems.

- **Sleep Disturbances:** Stress often interferes with sleep patterns, leading to insomnia, poor-quality sleep, and fatigue.

- **Hormonal Imbalance:** Chronic stress can disrupt the endocrine system, affecting hormonal balance and potentially leading to issues like weight gain and metabolic disorders.

Mental and Emotional Effects of Stress

- **Anxiety and Depression:** Chronic stress is a significant risk factor for mental health conditions such as anxiety and depression, often exacerbating symptoms.

- **Cognitive Impairment:** Prolonged stress can affect memory, concentration, and decision-making abilities, making it difficult to focus and think clearly.

- **Emotional Instability:** Stress can lead to mood swings, irritability, and a sense of overwhelm, affecting relationships and overall emotional well-being.

The Importance of Stress Management

Given the pervasive impact of stress on health, effective stress management is essential for maintaining well-being. Managing stress not only improves physical health but also enhances mental clarity, emotional stability, and overall life satisfaction.

Enhancing Physical Health

- **Improving Immune Function:** By managing stress, the immune system can function more effectively, reducing the frequency and severity of illnesses.

- **Supporting Heart Health:** Effective stress management techniques can lower blood pressure and reduce the risk of cardiovascular diseases.

- **Promoting Digestive Health:** Managing stress can alleviate digestive problems and promote better absorption of nutrients, contributing to overall wellness.

- **Better Sleep Quality:** Reducing stress can lead to more restful and rejuvenating sleep, which is vital for physical recovery and mental health.

Boosting Mental and Emotional Well-Being

- **Reducing Anxiety and Depression:** Effective stress management can lower the risk of developing anxiety and depression, providing a more stable and positive emotional state.

- **Improving Cognitive Function:** Managing stress helps maintain cognitive abilities, improving focus, memory, and decision-making skills.

- **Fostering Emotional Resilience:** Stress management techniques help build emotional resilience, enabling individuals to cope better with life's challenges.

Effective Stress Management Techniques

Managing stress involves both short-term strategies for immediate relief and long-term practices that build resilience and reduce stress over time.

Short-Term Stress Relief Techniques

- **Deep Breathing Exercises:** Simple deep breathing exercises can help calm the nervous system and reduce stress quickly. Techniques like diaphragmatic breathing or the 4-7-8 method are particularly effective.

- **Mindfulness and Meditation:** Mindfulness involves focusing on the present moment without judgment. Meditation practices like guided imagery, mindfulness meditation, or progressive muscle relaxation can quickly reduce stress levels.

- **Physical Activity:** Engaging in physical activity, even for a short period, can help lower cortisol levels and release endorphins, the body's natural stress relievers.

- **Aromatherapy:** Using essential oils like lavender, chamomile, or eucalyptus in diffusers or during massage can create a calming environment and help reduce stress.

Long-Term Stress Management Strategies

- **Regular Exercise:** Consistent physical activity is one of the most effective ways to manage stress. Exercise not only improves physical health but also releases endorphins, which enhance mood and reduce stress.

- **Healthy Diet:** A balanced diet rich in whole foods supports the body's ability to handle stress. Nutrient-dense foods can stabilize blood sugar levels, reducing mood swings and energy crashes that can contribute to stress.

- **Adequate Sleep:** Prioritizing sleep and maintaining a consistent sleep schedule helps the body recover from stress and prepare for the challenges of the next day.

- **Social Support:** Building and maintaining strong relationships with family, friends, and community provides emotional support during stressful times. Social interactions can help buffer the effects of stress and provide a sense of belonging.

- **Time Management:** Effective time management reduces the feeling of being overwhelmed. Prioritizing tasks, setting realistic goals, and taking breaks can prevent burnout and reduce stress.

- **Relaxation Techniques:** Incorporating relaxation techniques like yoga, tai chi, or deep relaxation exercises into daily routines can help lower stress levels over time.

Incorporating Stress Management into Daily Life

Incorporating stress management techniques into daily routines is essential for long-term well-being. Here are some practical ways to make stress management a part of everyday life:

- **Create a Routine:** Establish a daily routine that includes time for stress-relief activities such as exercise, meditation, or hobbies.

- **Set Boundaries:** Learn to say no and set boundaries to avoid overcommitting and becoming overwhelmed.

- **Practice Gratitude:** Regularly practicing gratitude can shift focus away from stressors and promote a positive outlook on life.

- **Stay Connected:** Maintain regular contact with supportive people who can provide encouragement and perspective during stressful times.

Stress management is a vital component of overall well-being, impacting both physical and mental health. By understanding the effects of stress and implementing effective management techniques, individuals can improve their quality of life, enhance resilience, and promote long-term health. Incorporating stress management practices into daily life not only reduces the immediate effects of stress but also builds a foundation for a healthier and more balanced life.

Techniques for Relaxation and Mental Clarity

In today's fast-paced world, finding moments of relaxation and mental clarity can be challenging. However, incorporating specific techniques into daily life can greatly enhance well-being, reduce stress, and improve cognitive function. These practices not only help to unwind but also foster a deeper sense of peace and focus, contributing to overall mental and physical health.

The Importance of Relaxation and Mental Clarity

Relaxation is essential for reducing the physical and emotional effects of stress, allowing the body to recover and rejuvenate. Mental clarity, on the other hand, involves maintaining a sharp, focused, and calm mind, which is crucial for decision-making, problem-solving, and overall cognitive function.

- **Physical Benefits:** Relaxation helps lower blood pressure, reduce muscle tension, and improve sleep quality. It also supports immune function by reducing the stress hormone cortisol.

- **Mental Benefits:** Techniques that promote mental clarity enhance concentration, memory, and creativity. They also help in managing anxiety, depression, and other mental health issues.

- **Emotional Benefits:** Relaxation techniques can lead to improved mood, greater emotional stability, and a more positive outlook on life.

Techniques for Relaxation

There are various techniques to promote relaxation, each offering unique benefits. Integrating these practices into your routine can help you achieve a state of calm and reduce the impact of daily stressors.

1. Deep Breathing Exercises

Deep breathing exercises are one of the simplest and most effective ways to induce relaxation. By focusing on slow, deep breaths, you can activate the body's relaxation response, reducing stress and anxiety.

- **Diaphragmatic Breathing:** Also known as belly breathing, this technique involves breathing deeply into the diaphragm rather than the chest. Place one hand on your stomach and the other on your chest, then breathe in deeply through your nose, ensuring your stomach rises while your chest remains still. Exhale slowly through your mouth.

- **4-7-8 Breathing:** Inhale quietly through your nose for a count of 4, hold your breath for a count of 7, and exhale completely through your mouth for a count of 8. Repeat this cycle several times to calm the nervous system.

2. Progressive Muscle Relaxation

Progressive muscle relaxation involves tensing and then slowly releasing each muscle group in the body. This technique helps to release physical tension and promote a state of deep relaxation.

- **Step-by-Step Process:** Start by tensing the muscles in your toes for a few seconds and then slowly releasing them. Gradually work your way up through the muscle groups in your legs, abdomen, chest, arms, and finally your face.

- **Mind-Body Connection:** Focus on the sensation of relaxation that follows each release of tension, which helps to heighten awareness of physical stress and encourage mental calmness.

3. Visualization and Guided Imagery

Visualization techniques involve creating mental images that promote calmness and relaxation. Guided imagery takes this a step further by following a narrated guide through a calming scenario.

- **Creating a Safe Space:** Close your eyes and imagine a peaceful, serene place where you feel safe and relaxed. This could be a beach, a forest, or any location that brings you comfort.

- **Engage the Senses:** Visualize the details of this place—what you see, hear, smell, and feel. Engaging all your senses in this mental imagery can deepen the relaxation experience.

4. Aromatherapy

Aromatherapy uses essential oils to promote relaxation and well-being. The inhalation of certain scents can trigger relaxation responses in the brain.

- **Lavender:** Known for its calming properties, lavender is often used to reduce anxiety and promote sleep.

- **Chamomile:** Chamomile is soothing and can help with stress reduction and relaxation.

- **Eucalyptus:** This oil is refreshing and can help clear the mind, making it easier to relax and focus.

5. Mindful Walking

Mindful walking involves walking slowly and deliberately, focusing on the movement of your body and your surroundings. This practice can be done indoors or outdoors and helps in grounding your mind and body.

- **Focus on Movement:** Pay attention to how your feet touch the ground, the rhythm of your steps, and the movement of your body. This focus helps to clear the mind and reduce stress.

- **Engage with the Environment:** Notice the sounds, sights, and smells around you as you walk. This connection with your environment can enhance the calming effects of the walk.

Techniques for Mental Clarity

Mental clarity involves having a clear and focused mind, which is essential for productivity, creativity, and effective decision-making. These techniques can help in achieving and maintaining mental clarity.

1. Mindfulness Meditation

Mindfulness meditation is the practice of focusing your attention on the present moment without judgment. It helps to reduce mental clutter and enhances clarity and focus.

- **Basic Practice:** Sit quietly and focus on your breath. If your mind starts to wander, gently bring your focus back to your breathing. The key is to observe your thoughts without getting attached to them.

- **Daily Practice:** Consistently practicing mindfulness meditation, even for just a few minutes a day, can significantly improve mental clarity and reduce stress.

2. Journaling

Journaling is a powerful tool for clearing the mind and gaining insight into your thoughts and feelings. Writing down your thoughts can help organize your mind and provide clarity on issues that may be troubling you.

- **Morning Pages:** A popular method involves writing three pages of free-form thoughts first thing in the morning. This practice helps to clear mental clutter and set a focused tone for the day.

- **Reflective Journaling:** Writing about your day, thoughts, and feelings before bed can help process emotions and clear your mind for better sleep and mental clarity.

3. Brain Dump

A brain dump is a simple technique where you write down everything that's on your mind, without worrying about organization or structure. This helps to relieve mental overload and clarify your thoughts.

- **Frequent Use:** Use a brain dump whenever you feel overwhelmed by thoughts or tasks. This can help declutter your mind and make it easier to prioritize and focus.

- **Categorization:** After dumping your thoughts onto paper, you can categorize and prioritize them, which helps in creating a clear action plan.

4. Pomodoro Technique

The Pomodoro Technique is a time management method that helps maintain focus and mental clarity. It involves working for 25-minute intervals followed by a 5-minute break.

- **Focused Work:** During each 25-minute session (called a Pomodoro), focus on one task without distractions. This helps maintain mental clarity and productivity.

- **Regular Breaks:** The short breaks help to refresh your mind, preventing mental fatigue and maintaining clarity throughout the day.

5. Decluttering Your Environment

A cluttered environment can lead to a cluttered mind. Keeping your physical space organized and tidy can enhance mental clarity and focus.

- **Workspace Organization:** Keep your desk and workspace clean and organized to reduce distractions and promote a clear mind.

- **Minimalism:** Embrace a minimalist approach to your living space, reducing unnecessary items that can contribute to mental clutter.

Integrating Relaxation and Mental Clarity Techniques into Daily Life

Incorporating these techniques into your daily routine can help create a balanced and harmonious life.

- **Routine Practices:** Set aside specific times each day for relaxation and mental clarity exercises, such as meditation in the morning or deep breathing before bed.

- **Mindful Transitions:** Use transition periods between tasks or at the end of the day to practice quick relaxation techniques like deep breathing or visualization.

- **Consistency:** The key to benefiting from these techniques is consistency. Regular practice leads to lasting results, enhancing overall well-being.

Techniques for relaxation and mental clarity are essential tools in managing stress and maintaining a healthy mind and body. By integrating these practices into daily life, you can cultivate a state of calm, improve cognitive function, and enhance overall well-being. Whether through deep breathing, mindfulness meditation, or decluttering your environment, these techniques offer a pathway to a more peaceful and focused life.

Incorporating Mindfulness and Meditation into Daily Life

Incorporating mindfulness and meditation into daily life can transform how we interact with the world and ourselves. These practices, rooted in ancient traditions, have gained significant attention in modern times for their profound effects on mental and physical well-being. By making mindfulness and meditation a regular part of your routine, you can cultivate greater awareness, reduce stress, and improve overall life satisfaction.

The Importance of Mindfulness and Meditation

Mindfulness involves paying attention to the present moment without judgment, while meditation is a practice that often involves focusing the mind to achieve a state of mental clarity and emotional calmness. Both practices are interrelated and offer numerous benefits:

- **Stress Reduction:** Regular mindfulness and meditation practice lowers cortisol levels, the hormone associated with stress, helping to reduce anxiety and promote relaxation.

- **Improved Focus and Concentration:** Mindfulness helps in training the brain to stay focused on the present, improving attention span and cognitive performance.

- **Emotional Regulation:** These practices enhance self-awareness and emotional regulation, allowing individuals to respond to situations with greater calmness and clarity.

- **Physical Health Benefits:** Meditation and mindfulness have been linked to lower blood pressure, improved immune function, and better sleep quality.

Getting Started with Mindfulness and Meditation

For those new to mindfulness and meditation, starting can seem daunting. However, the beauty of these practices lies in their simplicity and adaptability to any lifestyle.

1. Start Small

- **Short Sessions:** Begin with just a few minutes each day. Even five minutes of focused breathing or meditation can make a difference.

- **Consistency:** It's more important to practice regularly than to practice for long periods. Aim to incorporate mindfulness into your daily routine rather than focusing on the duration.

2. Choose a Comfortable Space

- **Quiet Environment:** Find a quiet, comfortable place where you won't be disturbed. This helps in creating a peaceful atmosphere conducive to meditation.

- **Comfortable Position:** Sit or lie down in a comfortable position. Whether you're sitting cross-legged on a cushion, lying down, or sitting in a chair, ensure your posture is relaxed yet alert.

Mindfulness Techniques for Daily Life

Mindfulness can be practiced anytime, anywhere. Here are some techniques to integrate mindfulness into your daily activities:

1. Mindful Breathing

- **Focus on the Breath:** Pay attention to your breathing without trying to change it. Notice the sensation of the air entering and leaving your nostrils, the rise and fall of your chest, or the feeling of your belly expanding and contracting.

- **Anchor Yourself:** Use your breath as an anchor whenever your mind starts to wander. Bringing attention back to your breath helps center your thoughts and maintain focus.

2. Mindful Eating

- **Savor Each Bite:** Slow down and pay full attention to the process of eating. Notice the colors, smells, textures, and flavors of your food.

- **Chew Slowly:** Chew each bite thoroughly and appreciate the taste and texture. This practice not only enhances digestion but also fosters a deeper connection with the act of nourishing your body.

3. Mindful Walking

- **Awareness of Movement:** Whether you're walking to work, through a park, or just around your home, focus on the sensation of your feet touching the ground, the rhythm of your steps, and the movement of your body.

- **Connection with Surroundings:** Notice your surroundings, the sounds, smells, and sights around you. This practice helps you stay grounded and connected to the present moment.

4. Mindful Listening

- **Active Listening:** When engaging in conversation, listen fully to the other person without planning your response. Focus on their words, tone, and body language.

- **Non-Judgmental Awareness:** Try to listen without immediately labeling or judging what is being said. This helps in building better communication and deeper connections.

Meditation Techniques for Daily Life

Meditation involves setting aside time to focus the mind and cultivate inner peace. There are various meditation techniques, each with unique benefits.

1. Focused Attention Meditation

- **Single Point of Focus:** Choose an object of focus, such as your breath, a mantra, or a candle flame. Keep your attention on this point, gently bringing your mind back whenever it wanders.

- **Regular Practice:** Start with short sessions of 5-10 minutes, gradually increasing the duration as you become more comfortable with the practice.

2. Loving-Kindness Meditation (Metta)

- **Cultivate Compassion:** Begin by focusing on yourself, repeating phrases like "May I be happy, may I be healthy, may I be at peace." Gradually extend these wishes to others— loved ones, acquaintances, and even those with whom you have conflict.

- **Expand the Circle:** As you practice, widen the circle of loving-kindness to include all living beings, fostering a sense of compassion and connection with the world.

3. Body Scan Meditation

- **Mindful Awareness of the Body:** Starting from the top of your head, slowly move your attention down through your body, noticing any sensations, tensions, or areas of relaxation.

- **Release Tension:** As you become aware of tension in any part of your body, consciously relax those muscles, releasing any tightness or discomfort.

4. Guided Meditation

- **Using Technology:** Utilize apps, online videos, or recordings where a guide takes you through a meditation session. This can be helpful for beginners who need structure and support in their practice.

- **Diverse Options:** There are guided meditations for various needs, such as relaxation, sleep, stress relief, and more. Choose the one that suits your current state of mind.

Integrating Mindfulness and Meditation into Your Routine

The key to reaping the benefits of mindfulness and meditation is consistent practice. Here are some tips for integrating these practices into your daily routine:

1. Set a Regular Time

- **Morning Practice:** Starting your day with mindfulness or meditation sets a positive tone for the rest of the day. It helps in grounding yourself before engaging with daily tasks.

- **Evening Wind-Down:** Practicing mindfulness or meditation in the evening can help in releasing the day's stress and preparing your mind and body for restful sleep.

2. Create Rituals

- **Mindful Morning Ritual:** Incorporate mindfulness into your morning routine, whether it's through mindful breathing while brushing your teeth or savoring your breakfast without distractions.

- **Evening Reflection:** Spend a few minutes each evening reflecting on your day. Focus on moments of gratitude or lessons learned, helping to cultivate a positive mindset.

3. Use Reminders

- **Mindfulness Cues:** Set reminders on your phone or place sticky notes around your home to prompt mindful moments throughout the day.

- **Routine Activities:** Pair mindfulness with daily activities, such as taking a mindful breath every time you sit down or stand up.

Overcoming Challenges

Incorporating mindfulness and meditation into daily life can come with challenges, especially for beginners. Here are some common obstacles and how to overcome them:

1. Dealing with a Busy Mind

- **Gentle Redirection:** It's natural for the mind to wander during mindfulness or meditation. Instead of getting frustrated, gently guide your focus back to your breath or point of meditation.

- **Practice Patience:** Developing mental stillness takes time. Be patient with yourself and acknowledge that it's okay to have an active mind.

2. Finding Time

- **Short Sessions:** If time is a constraint, start with short sessions. Even a few minutes of mindfulness or meditation can be beneficial.

- **Integrate into Daily Life:** Practice mindfulness during routine activities, such as mindful walking to work or mindful eating during meals.

3. Managing Expectations

- **Let Go of Perfection:** Understand that mindfulness and meditation are not about achieving a specific state but about being present and aware. Let go of expectations and simply experience the practice.

- **Celebrate Small Wins:** Acknowledge and appreciate the small moments of mindfulness and clarity you experience. Over time, these small wins contribute to overall well-being.

Incorporating mindfulness and meditation into daily life is a powerful way to cultivate inner peace, reduce stress, and enhance mental clarity. By starting small, choosing the right techniques, and integrating these practices into your routine, you can experience profound changes in your overall well-being. Remember, the journey is about consistent practice and embracing the present moment, leading to a more balanced, peaceful, and fulfilling life.

Chapter 3: S – Sleep

Understanding the Science of Sleep

Sleep is a vital biological process that plays a critical role in overall health and well-being. Despite its importance, sleep is often overlooked in favor of work, social activities, and entertainment. Understanding the science of sleep reveals why it is so essential and how it affects various aspects of our lives.

The Sleep Cycle

Sleep is not a uniform state; it is composed of multiple stages that cycle throughout the night. These stages can be broadly categorized into two main types:

1. **Non-Rapid Eye Movement (NREM) Sleep:**

   o **Stage 1:** This is the lightest stage of sleep, lasting just a few minutes. It's the transition between wakefulness and sleep, where the body begins to relax, and brain activity slows down.

   o **Stage 2:** In this stage, heart rate slows, and body temperature drops. Brain activity continues to decrease, but short bursts of rapid activity, known as sleep spindles, occur. This stage accounts for about 50% of the total sleep cycle.

   o **Stages 3:** This is the deepest stage of NREM sleep, often referred to as slow-wave sleep (SWS) or deep sleep. During this stage, the body repairs and regrows tissues, builds bone and muscle, and strengthens the immune system.

2. **Rapid Eye Movement (REM) Sleep:**

   o **REM Sleep:** This stage is characterized by rapid eye movements, increased brain activity, and vivid dreams. The body's muscles are temporarily paralyzed, preventing the sleeper from acting out dreams. REM sleep is crucial for cognitive functions such as memory consolidation, learning, and emotional regulation.

A full sleep cycle lasts about 90 minutes and repeats 4-6 times per night. The proportion of REM sleep increases with each cycle, making the last few hours of sleep particularly important for cognitive health.

The Role of Sleep in Physical Health

Sleep is essential for various physiological processes that keep the body functioning optimally.

1. **Tissue Repair and Growth:** During deep sleep, the body releases growth hormone, which is crucial for tissue repair and muscle growth. This stage is particularly important for athletes and those recovering from injuries.

2. **Immune Function:** Sleep is closely linked to the immune system. During sleep, the body produces cytokines, proteins that help fight infection, inflammation, and stress. Chronic sleep deprivation can weaken the immune response, making individuals more susceptible to illness.

3. **Metabolic Regulation:** Sleep affects the hormones that control hunger and satiety, such as ghrelin and leptin. Lack of sleep can lead to an imbalance in these hormones, increasing appetite and cravings for unhealthy foods, which may contribute to weight gain and obesity.

4. **Cardiovascular Health:** Adequate sleep helps maintain healthy blood pressure and reduces the risk of heart disease. During sleep, the heart rate and blood pressure decrease, giving the cardiovascular system a chance to rest and recover.

The Impact of Sleep on Cognitive Function

Sleep is crucial for brain health and cognitive function, influencing everything from memory to mood.

1. **Memory Consolidation:** During sleep, the brain processes and consolidates information learned throughout the day, transferring it from short-term to long-term memory. REM sleep is particularly important for this process.

2. **Learning and Problem-Solving:** Sleep enhances cognitive processes like learning, problem-solving, and creativity. It allows the brain to integrate and reorganize information, leading to better understanding and retention.

3. **Emotional Regulation:** Sleep plays a key role in regulating emotions. Lack of sleep can lead to irritability, mood swings, and increased susceptibility to stress. Chronic sleep deprivation is also linked to mental health disorders such as depression and anxiety.

4. **Attention and Concentration:** Adequate sleep is necessary for maintaining attention, concentration, and reaction times. Sleep-deprived individuals often struggle with focus, decision-making, and performing complex tasks.

The Effects of Sleep Deprivation

Chronic sleep deprivation can have serious consequences for both physical and mental health.

1. **Impaired Cognitive Function:** Lack of sleep impairs cognitive abilities, including memory, attention, and decision-making. It can lead to decreased productivity, errors at work, and a higher risk of accidents.

2. **Increased Risk of Chronic Diseases:** Sleep deprivation is associated with a higher risk of chronic conditions such as hypertension, diabetes, heart disease, and stroke. It also weakens the immune system, making the body more vulnerable to infections.

3. **Mood Disturbances:** Sleep deprivation can lead to irritability, anxiety, and depression. It affects the brain's ability to regulate emotions, leading to mood swings and increased stress levels.

4. **Weight Gain:** Lack of sleep disrupts the balance of hunger hormones, leading to increased appetite and cravings for high-calorie, sugary foods. This can contribute to weight gain and obesity over time.

5. **Decreased Quality of Life:** Chronic sleep deprivation affects overall quality of life, leading to fatigue, reduced energy levels, and decreased enjoyment of daily activities.

Factors Affecting Sleep Quality

Several factors can influence the quality of sleep, including lifestyle, environment, and health conditions.

1. **Sleep Environment:** A conducive sleep environment is essential for good sleep quality. Factors such as noise, light, temperature, and comfort of the mattress and pillows can all impact sleep.

2. **Lifestyle Habits:** Habits such as irregular sleep schedules, excessive caffeine or alcohol consumption, and lack of physical activity can disrupt sleep patterns. Establishing a regular sleep routine and practicing good sleep hygiene can improve sleep quality.

3. **Stress and Anxiety:** High levels of stress and anxiety can interfere with the ability to fall asleep and stay asleep. Practicing relaxation techniques, such as meditation or deep breathing, can help calm the mind and promote better sleep.

4. **Medical Conditions:** Conditions such as sleep apnea, restless leg syndrome, and chronic pain can significantly affect sleep quality. It's important to address any underlying health issues that may be disrupting sleep.

5. **Technology Use:** The use of electronic devices before bedtime can interfere with sleep. The blue light emitted by screens suppresses melatonin production, making it harder to fall asleep. Limiting screen time before bed and creating a technology-free sleep environment can improve sleep quality.

Strategies for Improving Sleep

Improving sleep quality involves adopting healthy sleep habits and addressing factors that may be disrupting sleep.

1. **Establish a Sleep Routine:** Go to bed and wake up at the same time every day, even on weekends. This helps regulate the body's internal clock and improves sleep consistency.

2. **Create a Relaxing Bedtime Routine:** Engage in relaxing activities before bed, such as reading, taking a warm bath, or practicing relaxation techniques. This helps signal to the body that it's time to wind down.

3. **Optimize the Sleep Environment:** Ensure the sleep environment is conducive to rest. Keep the bedroom dark, quiet, and cool, and invest in a comfortable mattress and pillows.

4. **Limit Caffeine and Alcohol:** Avoid consuming caffeine and alcohol in the hours leading up to bedtime, as they can interfere with sleep. Opt for herbal teas or other non-caffeinated beverages instead.

5. **Stay Active:** Regular physical activity promotes better sleep, but it's important to avoid vigorous exercise close to bedtime, as it may have a stimulating effect.

6. **Manage Stress:** Practice stress management techniques, such as meditation, deep breathing, or yoga, to calm the mind and reduce anxiety that may interfere with sleep.

7. **Limit Screen Time:** Avoid using electronic devices at least an hour before bed. If you must use a screen, consider using a blue light filter to reduce its impact on sleep.

8. **Consider Sleep Aids:** If necessary, natural sleep aids such as melatonin supplements or herbal teas like chamomile can help promote sleep. However, it's important to consult a healthcare provider before using any sleep aids.

Understanding the science of sleep highlights its crucial role in overall health and well-being. By prioritizing sleep and adopting healthy sleep habits, individuals can improve not only their physical health but also their mental and emotional well-being. Quality sleep is a cornerstone of a healthy lifestyle, and investing in good sleep practices is an investment in long-term health and vitality.

Creating Healthy Sleep Habits for Restorative Rest

Restorative sleep is essential for physical and mental well-being. It's not just about the quantity of sleep but also the quality that matters. Creating healthy sleep habits can transform your sleep patterns, leading to more restorative rest and overall better health.

Establishing a Consistent Sleep Schedule

One of the most effective ways to improve sleep quality is by maintaining a consistent sleep schedule. The body's internal clock, or circadian rhythm, thrives on regularity. Going to bed and waking up at the same time every day, even on weekends, helps regulate this rhythm, making it easier to fall asleep and wake up naturally.

Steps to Establish a Consistent Sleep Schedule:

1. **Set a Fixed Bedtime and Wake-Up Time:** Choose a bedtime that allows for 7-9 hours of sleep and stick to it. Set an alarm for the same wake-up time every day, including weekends.

2. **Gradually Adjust Your Schedule:** If your current sleep schedule is erratic, gradually shift your bedtime and wake-up time by 15-30 minutes earlier or later each day until you reach your desired schedule.

3. **Avoid Napping Late in the Day:** If you nap, keep it short (20-30 minutes) and avoid napping late in the afternoon or evening, as this can interfere with nighttime sleep.

Creating a Sleep-Inducing Environment

The environment in which you sleep plays a significant role in the quality of your rest. A comfortable, quiet, and dark room can enhance sleep by minimizing disruptions.

Tips for Creating a Sleep-Inducing Environment:

1. **Keep Your Bedroom Cool:** The ideal room temperature for sleep is between 60-67°F (15-19°C). A cool room promotes the natural drop in body temperature that occurs during sleep.

2. **Reduce Noise:** Use earplugs, a white noise machine, or a fan to block out disruptive noises. Soft, consistent sounds can drown out sudden noises that might wake you.

3. **Darken the Room:** Darkness signals the body to produce melatonin, a hormone that induces sleep. Use blackout curtains or a sleep mask to block out light from windows, and eliminate or cover light sources from electronic devices.

4. **Invest in Comfortable Bedding:** A supportive mattress and pillows tailored to your sleeping position can prevent discomfort and improve sleep quality. Choose breathable, natural fabrics for sheets and blankets to enhance comfort.

5. **Minimize Electronic Devices:** Remove or turn off electronic devices like TVs, computers, and smartphones from the bedroom. The blue light emitted by screens can interfere with melatonin production and disrupt sleep.

Developing a Relaxing Bedtime Routine

A calming pre-sleep routine can signal to your body that it's time to wind down, making it easier to transition from wakefulness to sleep.

Suggestions for a Relaxing Bedtime Routine:

1. **Engage in Relaxing Activities:** Spend the last hour before bed doing activities that relax you, such as reading a book, listening to soothing music, or taking a warm bath.

2. **Practice Relaxation Techniques:** Techniques like deep breathing, progressive muscle relaxation, or gentle yoga can help reduce tension and prepare your body for sleep.

3. **Avoid Stimulating Activities:** Avoid activities that can be stimulating, such as intense exercise, heavy meals, or emotionally charged conversations, in the hour leading up to bedtime.

4. **Limit Exposure to Screens:** Reduce screen time before bed to prevent the blue light from interfering with your body's sleep-wake cycle. Instead, opt for low-light activities like reading a physical book or journaling.

Mindful Eating and Drinking Before Bed

What you consume in the hours leading up to bedtime can significantly impact your sleep quality. Mindful eating and drinking can help prevent disruptions during the night.

Guidelines for Eating and Drinking Before Bed:

1. **Avoid Heavy Meals:** Eating large, heavy meals close to bedtime can cause discomfort and indigestion, making it harder to fall asleep. Try to have dinner at least 2-3 hours before bedtime.

2. **Limit Caffeine and Alcohol:** Caffeine is a stimulant that can stay in your system for hours, so it's best to avoid it in the afternoon and evening. While alcohol may make you feel sleepy

initially, it can disrupt sleep later in the night, so limit consumption, especially close to bedtime.

3. **Stay Hydrated:** While it's important to stay hydrated, drinking too much liquid before bed can lead to frequent trips to the bathroom, disrupting sleep. Try to drink the majority of your fluids earlier in the day.

Physical Activity and Its Timing

Regular physical activity is beneficial for sleep, but timing is crucial. Exercise can help you fall asleep faster and enjoy deeper sleep, but it's important to consider when you're working out.

How to Incorporate Physical Activity for Better Sleep:

1. **Exercise Earlier in the Day:** Engage in vigorous exercise earlier in the day to give your body enough time to wind down before bed. Morning or early afternoon workouts are ideal.

2. **Try Gentle Evening Activities:** If you prefer exercising in the evening, opt for light activities such as stretching, walking, or yoga. These activities can help relax your body and mind without overstimulating your system.

3. **Listen to Your Body:** Everyone's body responds differently to exercise, so pay attention to how your workouts affect your sleep and adjust your routine accordingly.

Managing Stress and Anxiety for Better Sleep

Stress and anxiety are common culprits of sleep disturbances. Developing strategies to manage stress can significantly improve your ability to fall asleep and stay asleep.

Strategies for Managing Stress and Anxiety:

1. **Practice Mindfulness and Meditation:** Mindfulness practices and meditation can help calm the mind, reduce anxiety, and create a sense of peace that is conducive to sleep.

2. **Write Down Your Worries:** If you find yourself lying awake worrying about the next day, try writing down your thoughts and creating a to-do list before bed. This can help clear your mind and prevent overthinking during the night.

3. **Focus on Relaxation:** Incorporate relaxation techniques such as deep breathing, visualization, or progressive muscle relaxation into your bedtime routine to release physical and mental tension.

4. **Create a Worry Time:** Designate a specific time earlier in the day to address any concerns or worries. By dealing with these issues before bedtime, you can prevent them from disrupting your sleep.

The Role of Sleep Hygiene

Sleep hygiene refers to the habits and practices that promote consistent, quality sleep. Good sleep hygiene is the foundation for achieving restorative rest.

Essential Sleep Hygiene Practices:

1. **Limit Naps:** While short naps can be refreshing, long or irregular napping during the day can negatively affect nighttime sleep. If you need to nap, keep it brief and early in the afternoon.

2. **Wake Up to Natural Light:** Exposure to natural light in the morning helps regulate your circadian rhythm. Try to spend time outside in the morning or keep your blinds open to let in sunlight.

3. **Stick to a Routine:** Consistency in your daily routine helps your body recognize when it's time to sleep. Try to follow a similar schedule every day, even on weekends.

4. **Avoid Clock-Watching:** Constantly checking the clock when you can't sleep can increase anxiety and make it harder to drift off. If you can't sleep, get out of bed and do something relaxing until you feel sleepy.

Creating healthy sleep habits is a powerful way to achieve restorative rest and enhance your overall well-being. By establishing a consistent sleep schedule, creating a sleep-inducing environment, developing a relaxing bedtime routine, and practicing good sleep hygiene, you can improve the quality of your sleep and wake up feeling refreshed and rejuvenated. Prioritizing sleep as an essential part of your daily routine is an investment in your health, energy, and longevity.

The Connection Between Sleep and Immune Function

Sleep is not just a time for rest and recovery; it plays a critical role in maintaining and boosting the immune system. The connection between sleep and immune function is profound, influencing everything from the body's ability to fight infections to its response to vaccinations. Understanding this relationship highlights the importance of prioritizing good sleep habits as a cornerstone of overall health and disease prevention.

The Immune System: An Overview

The immune system is a complex network of cells, tissues, and organs that work together to defend the body against harmful invaders like bacteria, viruses, and other pathogens. It operates on two levels:

1. **Innate Immunity:** This is the body's first line of defense, responding quickly to infections with a general attack on invaders.

2. **Adaptive Immunity:** This is a more specialized response, where the body recognizes and remembers specific pathogens, allowing for a stronger and faster response upon future exposure.

Both innate and adaptive immunity are influenced by sleep, as sufficient rest is necessary for these systems to function optimally.

How Sleep Affects Immune Function

1. **Production of Immune Cells:** During sleep, particularly deep sleep (also known as slow-wave sleep), the body produces and releases cytokines. These are proteins that help regulate immune responses, including inflammation. Cytokines are crucial in fighting off infections and inflammation, and their production is increased during sleep.

2. **Memory Consolidation of the Immune System:** Just as sleep helps consolidate memories in the brain, it also aids the immune system in "remembering" pathogens. This is part of the adaptive immune system's function, where it learns to recognize and respond more

effectively to pathogens it has encountered before. Without sufficient sleep, this memory consolidation process is weakened, making the immune system less effective.

3. **Regulation of Inflammatory Responses:** Sleep helps regulate inflammation, a natural response of the immune system to infections or injuries. Chronic sleep deprivation can lead to an imbalance in this regulation, resulting in increased inflammation, which is associated with various chronic diseases such as heart disease, diabetes, and autoimmune disorders.

4. **Impact on Natural Killer Cells:** Natural killer (NK) cells are a type of white blood cell that play a crucial role in the early defense against viruses and tumors. Sleep deprivation has been shown to reduce the activity of NK cells, making the body more susceptible to infections and even cancer.

5. **Impact on Vaccination Response:** Sleep can also affect how well the body responds to vaccinations. Studies have shown that individuals who are sleep-deprived produce fewer antibodies in response to vaccines, which can decrease the effectiveness of the vaccination. Ensuring adequate sleep before and after receiving a vaccine can enhance the body's immune response.

Sleep and the Stress-Immune Connection

Chronic sleep deprivation can lead to increased levels of stress hormones like cortisol. Elevated cortisol levels can suppress immune function, reducing the body's ability to fight off infections. This creates a vicious cycle where lack of sleep increases stress, which in turn further weakens the immune system. Managing stress through adequate sleep is therefore essential for maintaining a strong immune defense.

Sleep Deprivation and Susceptibility to Illness

Lack of sleep can significantly increase susceptibility to illness. Research has shown that individuals who do not get enough sleep are more likely to catch colds and other infections. One study found that people who sleep less than six hours a night are four times more likely to catch a cold than those who sleep seven hours or more. This is because sleep deprivation lowers the body's ability to produce cytokines and other infection-fighting molecules.

The Role of Sleep in Recovery from Illness

Sleep is crucial for recovery when the body is fighting an infection. During sleep, the body can devote more energy to the immune system, helping to repair damage and fight off invaders. Fever, which is part of the immune response to infection, often spikes during sleep, helping the body to combat pathogens more effectively. This is why rest and sleep are often prescribed as part of the treatment for many illnesses.

Optimizing Sleep for a Healthy Immune System

Given the strong connection between sleep and immune function, it's important to adopt habits that promote healthy sleep. Here are some tips:

1. **Prioritize Sleep Duration:** Aim for 7-9 hours of sleep each night. This duration allows for complete sleep cycles, including stages of deep sleep that are essential for immune function.

2. **Maintain Sleep Quality:** Ensure your sleep is uninterrupted and restful. Avoid heavy meals, caffeine, and screens before bed, as these can disrupt sleep quality.

3. **Follow a Consistent Sleep Schedule:** Going to bed and waking up at the same time every day helps regulate your body's internal clock, supporting a strong immune system.

4. **Create a Sleep-Inducing Environment:** Keep your bedroom cool, dark, and quiet, and use a comfortable mattress and pillows to support quality sleep.

5. **Practice Stress Management:** Since stress can negatively impact both sleep and immune function, incorporate relaxation techniques such as mindfulness, meditation, or gentle yoga into your daily routine.

6. **Listen to Your Body:** Pay attention to your body's signals. If you're feeling run down, allow yourself extra rest to support your immune system.

Sleep is a fundamental component of a healthy immune system. By understanding the connection between sleep and immune function, we can appreciate the importance of prioritizing good sleep habits. Adequate and quality sleep not only helps in preventing infections and illnesses but also enhances the body's ability to recover from them. Embracing a lifestyle that supports restorative sleep is a powerful way to strengthen immunity and promote long-term health.

Chapter 4: T - Toxin Elimination

Detoxifying Your Body Naturally

Detoxification, or detox, is the body's natural process of eliminating toxins and harmful substances. Our bodies are exposed to various toxins daily, from environmental pollutants to processed foods and chemicals in personal care products. Detoxification is crucial for maintaining overall health and preventing chronic diseases. By supporting your body's natural detoxification processes, you can enhance your well-being, boost energy levels, and improve your immune system.

The Body's Natural Detoxification System

The human body has a sophisticated system designed to detoxify itself. The liver, kidneys, lungs, skin, and digestive system work together to neutralize and eliminate toxins. Here's how each organ contributes to detoxification:

1. **Liver:** The liver is the body's primary detoxification organ. It processes toxins and converts them into harmless substances or ones that can be excreted. The liver filters the blood, metabolizes drugs and alcohol, and produces bile to aid in digestion and the elimination of waste.

2. **Kidneys:** The kidneys filter blood and remove waste products and excess substances, which are then excreted as urine. They play a crucial role in maintaining the body's fluid and electrolyte balance, which is essential for detoxification.

3. **Lungs:** The lungs help expel toxins through respiration. They filter out volatile chemicals and expel carbon dioxide, a byproduct of cellular metabolism, from the body.

4. **Skin:** The skin is the body's largest organ and acts as a barrier to external toxins. It also eliminates toxins through sweat. Regular sweating through exercise or saunas can help remove impurities from the body.

5. **Digestive System:** The digestive system is responsible for processing food and eliminating waste. The intestines play a key role in absorbing nutrients and expelling toxins through bowel movements. A healthy gut microbiome supports efficient detoxification and overall health.

Natural Ways to Support Detoxification

While the body is equipped to detoxify itself, certain lifestyle choices and natural remedies can enhance this process. Here are some effective ways to support your body's natural detoxification:

1. **Stay Hydrated:** Water is essential for detoxification as it helps flush toxins out of the body through urine, sweat, and bowel movements. Drinking adequate water ensures that the kidneys function optimally and aids in digestion. Aim for at least 8-10 glasses of water daily, and consider starting your day with a glass of warm water with lemon to stimulate digestion and detoxification.

2. **Eat a Detoxifying Diet:** A diet rich in whole, unprocessed foods supports the body's detoxification processes. Focus on eating plenty of fruits, vegetables, whole grains, lean proteins, and healthy fats. Certain foods are particularly beneficial for detoxification:

   o **Cruciferous Vegetables:** Broccoli, cauliflower, and Brussels sprouts contain compounds that support liver detoxification.

   o **Leafy Greens:** Spinach, kale, and Swiss chard are high in chlorophyll, which helps neutralize toxins.

   o **Garlic and Onions:** These contain sulfur compounds that enhance liver function and support detoxification.

   o **Berries:** Blueberries, strawberries, and raspberries are rich in antioxidants that help neutralize free radicals and reduce oxidative stress.

   o **Citrus Fruits:** Lemons, oranges, and grapefruits are high in vitamin C, which boosts the immune system and supports detoxification.

3. **Limit Toxin Exposure:** Reducing your exposure to environmental toxins can significantly support your body's detoxification efforts. This includes avoiding processed foods, reducing the use of chemical-laden personal care products, and minimizing exposure to air pollution and household chemicals. Choose organic produce when possible to reduce pesticide intake and opt for natural cleaning products.

4. **Support Gut Health:** A healthy digestive system is crucial for detoxification. Consuming fiber-rich foods like fruits, vegetables, and whole grains helps maintain regular bowel movements, which are essential for eliminating waste. Probiotics and fermented foods like yogurt, kefir, and sauerkraut support a healthy gut microbiome, which plays a role in detoxification.

5. **Incorporate Herbs and Supplements:** Certain herbs and supplements can support the body's detoxification processes:

   o **Milk Thistle:** Known for its liver-protective properties, milk thistle helps regenerate liver cells and supports detoxification.

   o **Dandelion Root:** This herb acts as a diuretic, supporting kidney function and helping to flush out toxins through urine.

   o **Turmeric:** Turmeric contains curcumin, which has anti-inflammatory and antioxidant properties that support liver health.

   o **Cilantro:** This herb is believed to help remove heavy metals from the body, supporting overall detoxification.

6. **Exercise Regularly:** Physical activity is an excellent way to support detoxification. Exercise increases circulation, which helps transport toxins to the organs responsible for elimination. It also promotes sweating, which is another way the body expels toxins. Aim for at least 30 minutes of moderate exercise most days of the week, such as walking, jogging, or yoga.

7. **Get Adequate Sleep:** Sleep is essential for the body to repair and regenerate itself. During sleep, the brain clears out toxins that accumulate during the day. Prioritizing 7-9 hours of quality sleep each night supports overall health and detoxification.

8. **Practice Deep Breathing:** Deep breathing exercises can enhance lung function and support the body's natural detoxification. By taking slow, deep breaths, you increase oxygen intake and help expel carbon dioxide and other toxins. Incorporating deep breathing exercises into your daily routine can also reduce stress, which is beneficial for overall health.

9. **Try Dry Brushing:** Dry brushing is a technique that involves brushing the skin with a natural bristle brush in circular motions before showering. This practice stimulates the lymphatic system, which plays a key role in detoxification. Dry brushing also exfoliates the skin, removing dead cells and promoting circulation.

10. **Use Saunas or Steam Rooms:** Sweating is one of the body's natural ways to detoxify. Regular use of saunas or steam rooms can help remove toxins through sweat. The heat also promotes circulation and relaxation, supporting overall detoxification.

The Role of Mind-Body Practices in Detoxification

In addition to physical detoxification, it's important to consider the role of emotional and mental detoxification. Stress, negative emotions, and toxic relationships can have a significant impact on overall health. Incorporating mind-body practices like meditation, yoga, and mindfulness can help clear mental clutter, reduce stress, and support emotional detoxification.

Detoxifying your body naturally is not about drastic measures or extreme diets; it's about supporting your body's natural processes through a balanced lifestyle. By staying hydrated, eating a nutrient-rich diet, reducing toxin exposure, and incorporating natural remedies and practices, you can enhance your body's ability to detoxify and promote long-term health. Embracing these practices as part of your daily routine can lead to increased energy, improved immune function, and a greater sense of well-being.

The Role of Liver and Kidney Health in Detoxification

The liver and kidneys are two of the most vital organs in the body, playing central roles in the detoxification process. Their ability to filter, process, and eliminate toxins ensures that harmful substances are efficiently removed from the body, protecting overall health. Understanding how these organs work and how to support their function is essential for maintaining a healthy and effective detoxification system.

The Liver: The Body's Detox Powerhouse

The liver is the body's largest internal organ and a critical component of the detoxification system. It performs over 500 functions, many of which are directly related to detoxification, metabolism, and the regulation of various bodily processes.

Key Functions of the Liver in Detoxification:

1. **Filtering Blood:** The liver continuously filters the blood coming from the digestive tract before passing it to the rest of the body. During this process, the liver removes toxins, drugs, and waste products, converting them into less harmful substances.

2. **Metabolizing Toxins:** The liver uses a two-phase process to metabolize and neutralize toxins:

   o **Phase 1: Oxidation:** In this phase, enzymes in the liver (primarily cytochrome P450 enzymes) modify toxins, making them more water-soluble. This is necessary for the next step but can also create reactive intermediates, which are potentially harmful.

   o **Phase 2: Conjugation:** The liver attaches these reactive intermediates to other molecules, such as amino acids or sulfur-containing compounds, to neutralize them. These conjugated substances are now ready to be excreted from the body.

3. **Producing Bile:** The liver produces bile, a digestive fluid that plays a crucial role in the elimination of fat-soluble toxins and waste products. Bile binds to these substances in the intestines, allowing them to be excreted through feces.

4. **Regulating Metabolism:** The liver metabolizes nutrients and stores energy in the form of glycogen. It also breaks down and converts proteins, fats, and carbohydrates, which can help manage the body's energy needs and detoxify metabolic waste.

Supporting Liver Health:

To keep the liver functioning optimally, it's important to adopt lifestyle habits that support its health:

- **Maintain a Balanced Diet:** Eating a diet rich in antioxidants, vitamins, and minerals supports liver function. Foods like leafy greens, berries, and cruciferous vegetables (e.g., broccoli, Brussels sprouts) are particularly beneficial for the liver.

- **Limit Alcohol and Avoid Toxins:** Excessive alcohol consumption and exposure to environmental toxins can damage the liver. Reducing alcohol intake and avoiding harmful chemicals can help protect liver health.

- **Stay Hydrated:** Adequate water intake is essential for liver function as it helps flush out toxins and supports the body's metabolic processes.

- **Incorporate Liver-Supporting Herbs:** Herbs like milk thistle, dandelion root, and turmeric have been shown to support liver health and enhance its detoxification abilities.

The Kidneys: Filtering and Balancing the Body

The kidneys are another essential part of the body's detoxification system. These two bean-shaped organs are responsible for filtering blood, balancing fluids, and eliminating waste products through urine. The kidneys also play a role in regulating electrolytes, blood pressure, and the body's acid-base balance.

Key Functions of the Kidneys in Detoxification:

1. **Filtering Blood:** The kidneys filter about 120 to 150 quarts of blood daily, removing waste products and excess substances like urea, creatinine, and electrolytes. This filtration process produces about 1 to 2 quarts of urine, which carries waste out of the body.

2. **Eliminating Waste Products:** The kidneys remove metabolic waste products that are byproducts of normal cellular processes. This includes nitrogenous wastes, which are the result of protein metabolism.

3. **Balancing Electrolytes and Fluids:** The kidneys maintain the balance of electrolytes (such as sodium, potassium, and calcium) and ensure that the body has the right amount of fluid. This balance is crucial for the proper function of cells and organs and for the detoxification process.

4. **Regulating Blood Pressure:** The kidneys produce hormones that regulate blood pressure, which is important for ensuring adequate blood flow to the organs, including those involved in detoxification.

Supporting Kidney Health:

Just like the liver, the kidneys require care to function effectively:

- **Stay Hydrated:** Drinking plenty of water is essential for kidney health. Hydration helps the kidneys filter waste from the blood and prevents the formation of kidney stones.

- **Eat a Kidney-Friendly Diet:** Foods that support kidney health include those rich in antioxidants and anti-inflammatory properties, such as berries, leafy greens, and garlic. Reducing the intake of sodium, processed foods, and excessive protein can also help maintain kidney health.

- **Manage Blood Pressure:** Keeping blood pressure within a healthy range is crucial for kidney function. Regular physical activity, a balanced diet, and reducing stress can help manage blood pressure.

- **Limit Toxin Exposure:** Avoiding the overuse of medications that can be hard on the kidneys, such as nonsteroidal anti-inflammatory drugs (NSAIDs), and reducing exposure to environmental toxins can help protect the kidneys.

The Synergy Between Liver and Kidneys in Detoxification

The liver and kidneys work together in the detoxification process, each playing complementary roles. The liver metabolizes toxins, converting them into forms that can be easily excreted. Once these toxins are processed, the kidneys filter them out of the blood and eliminate them from the body through urine.

A holistic approach to detoxification involves supporting both the liver and kidneys through healthy lifestyle choices. By maintaining hydration, eating a nutrient-rich diet, avoiding harmful substances, and incorporating supportive herbs and practices, you can enhance the detoxification process and promote overall health and well-being.

The liver and kidneys are essential to the body's natural detoxification system. Understanding their roles and how to support them can help you maintain optimal health and protect your body from the harmful effects of toxins. By focusing on liver and kidney health through diet, hydration, and mindful living, you can enhance your body's ability to detoxify and sustain long-term wellness.

Using Herbs and Supplements to Support Detoxification

Herbs and supplements can play a significant role in supporting the body's natural detoxification processes. These natural remedies can help enhance liver and kidney function, aid in the removal of toxins, and improve overall health. By incorporating specific herbs and supplements into your daily routine, you can support your body's ability to detoxify effectively and maintain well-being.

Key Herbs for Detoxification

1. **Milk Thistle (Silybum marianum):** Milk thistle is one of the most well-known herbs for liver health. Its active component, silymarin, has antioxidant and anti-inflammatory properties that help protect liver cells from damage and support liver regeneration. Silymarin also aids in detoxification by enhancing the liver's ability to process and eliminate toxins.

   How to Use: Milk thistle can be taken in the form of capsules, tinctures, or teas. A typical dosage is 140-420 mg of silymarin per day.

2. **Dandelion Root (Taraxacum officinale):** Dandelion root is traditionally used as a diuretic and liver tonic. It helps increase urine production, supporting kidney function and the elimination of waste. Dandelion root also stimulates bile production, which aids in the digestion and removal of fats and toxins.

   How to Use: Dandelion root can be consumed as a tea, tincture, or in capsule form. The recommended dosage for dandelion root tea is 1-2 cups per day.

3. **Turmeric (Curcuma longa):** Turmeric contains curcumin, a compound with powerful anti-inflammatory and antioxidant properties. Curcumin supports liver function by reducing inflammation and oxidative stress, which can enhance the liver's ability to detoxify. It also aids in digestion and supports overall metabolic health.

   How to Use: Turmeric can be taken as a spice in food, in supplement form, or as a tea. For supplements, a typical dosage is 500-2000 mg of curcumin per day.

4. **Cilantro (Coriandrum sativum):** Cilantro is believed to help remove heavy metals from the body, such as mercury and lead. It contains compounds that can bind to heavy metals and support their excretion through the urine.

   How to Use: Cilantro can be added fresh to salads, smoothies, or used as a culinary herb. Cilantro supplements are also available, though they should be used with caution and under the guidance of a healthcare provider.

5. **Ginger (Zingiber officinale):** Ginger has anti-inflammatory and digestive-supporting properties. It can help stimulate digestion, improve gut health, and support the detoxification process by aiding in the elimination of waste and toxins.

   How to Use: Ginger can be consumed as a tea, added to food, or taken in supplement form. A typical dosage is 1-3 grams of ginger per day.

Key Supplements for Detoxification

1. **Activated Charcoal:** Activated charcoal is a form of carbon that has been treated to become highly porous, which helps it absorb toxins and chemicals. It can bind to a wide range of

substances, preventing their absorption in the gastrointestinal tract and aiding in their elimination.

How to Use: Activated charcoal is typically taken in capsule or powder form. The recommended dosage is 500-1000 mg before or between meals. It should be used with caution and not for prolonged periods, as it can interfere with nutrient absorption.

2. **N-acetylcysteine (NAC):** NAC is a precursor to glutathione, one of the body's most important antioxidants. It supports liver health by boosting glutathione levels, which helps neutralize free radicals and detoxify harmful substances.

How to Use: NAC is available in capsule or powder form. A typical dosage is 600-1200 mg per day.

3. **Milk Thistle Extract:** Besides being available as a whole herb, milk thistle can be taken in concentrated extract form. Milk thistle extract provides a higher dose of silymarin, which can be beneficial for those seeking additional liver support.

How to Use: Milk thistle extract supplements typically provide 70-80% silymarin. The recommended dosage is 140-420 mg of silymarin per day.

4. **Glutathione:** Glutathione is a potent antioxidant produced by the body that plays a critical role in detoxification. Supplementing with glutathione can help support liver function and improve the body's ability to neutralize and eliminate toxins.

How to Use: Glutathione supplements are available in oral, sublingual, and intravenous forms. The typical dosage is 250-500 mg per day for oral supplements.

5. **Spirulina:** Spirulina is a type of blue-green algae that is rich in nutrients and antioxidants. It supports liver and kidney health by providing essential vitamins and minerals that aid in detoxification.

How to Use: Spirulina is available in powder or tablet form. The recommended dosage is 1-3 grams per day.

Incorporating Herbs and Supplements into Your Routine

To effectively incorporate herbs and supplements into your detoxification regimen, consider the following tips:

1. **Consult a Healthcare Provider:** Before starting any new herbal or supplement regimen, consult with a healthcare provider, especially if you have underlying health conditions or are taking other medications.

2. **Start Slowly:** Begin with lower doses and gradually increase as needed. This approach allows you to monitor your body's response and adjust accordingly.

3. **Choose Quality Products:** Opt for high-quality, reputable brands to ensure the purity and efficacy of the herbs and supplements you use. Look for products that are standardized for active ingredients and free from contaminants.

4. **Monitor Your Health:** Keep track of any changes in your health and well-being. If you experience any adverse effects or discomfort, discontinue use and consult a healthcare provider.

5. **Combine with Healthy Lifestyle Choices:** Herbs and supplements should be used in conjunction with a balanced diet, regular exercise, and other healthy lifestyle practices to support overall detoxification and health.

Herbs and supplements can play a valuable role in supporting the body's natural detoxification processes. By incorporating specific herbs like milk thistle, dandelion root, and turmeric, along with supplements such as activated charcoal and NAC, you can enhance liver and kidney function, aid in toxin removal, and promote overall well-being. Always approach supplementation with care, and use these remedies as part of a holistic approach to health that includes a balanced diet and healthy lifestyle practices.

Chapter 5: A – Activity

The Benefits of Regular Physical Exercise

Regular physical exercise is a cornerstone of overall health and well-being. Engaging in consistent physical activity offers a wide array of benefits, ranging from improved cardiovascular health to enhanced mental clarity. This comprehensive look at the benefits of exercise will help you understand why making physical activity a regular part of your life is essential for maintaining optimal health.

1. Cardiovascular Health

Improved Heart Function: Regular exercise strengthens the heart muscle, improving its efficiency in pumping blood throughout the body. This enhances overall cardiovascular health, reduces the risk of heart disease, and helps manage blood pressure levels.

Reduced Risk of Heart Disease: Engaging in aerobic activities such as walking, running, or cycling lowers the risk of developing heart disease by improving cholesterol levels, reducing blood pressure, and decreasing inflammation.

Enhanced Circulation: Exercise promotes better blood flow and oxygen delivery to tissues and organs, supporting overall cardiovascular function and reducing the risk of vascular diseases.

2. Weight Management

Caloric Expenditure: Physical activity increases the number of calories burned, which helps in maintaining a healthy weight or losing excess weight. Combining regular exercise with a balanced diet can be an effective strategy for weight management.

Boosted Metabolism: Exercise boosts metabolic rate, which means that the body continues to burn calories at an elevated rate even after the workout is completed. This can help in preventing weight gain and maintaining a healthy body composition.

Reduced Body Fat: Regular exercise, especially resistance training, helps in reducing body fat by increasing muscle mass and improving overall body composition.

3. Musculoskeletal Health

Strengthened Muscles and Bones: Weight-bearing exercises such as strength training and resistance workouts enhance muscle strength and bone density. This is particularly important for preventing osteoporosis and reducing the risk of fractures as you age.

Improved Flexibility and Mobility: Regular stretching and dynamic exercises increase flexibility and range of motion, which can reduce the risk of injury and improve overall functional movement.

Enhanced Joint Health: Exercise helps in maintaining joint health by promoting the production of synovial fluid, which lubricates the joints and reduces stiffness.

4. Mental Health Benefits

Reduced Symptoms of Depression and Anxiety: Exercise stimulates the release of endorphins, which are natural mood elevators. Regular physical activity has been shown to reduce symptoms of depression and anxiety, leading to improved mental well-being.

Enhanced Cognitive Function: Physical activity improves brain function by increasing blood flow to the brain, which supports cognitive processes such as memory, attention, and learning. It also helps in reducing the risk of cognitive decline and neurodegenerative diseases.

Stress Reduction: Exercise acts as a natural stress reliever by lowering levels of the stress hormone cortisol and promoting relaxation. Engaging in physical activity can help manage daily stressors and enhance overall emotional resilience.

5. Enhanced Immune Function

Boosted Immune Response: Regular moderate exercise enhances the immune system's ability to fight off infections and diseases. It increases the circulation of immune cells in the body, helping to detect and respond to potential threats more effectively.

Reduced Inflammation: Exercise helps in reducing chronic inflammation, which is linked to various health conditions such as cardiovascular disease, diabetes, and certain cancers. By managing inflammation, exercise supports overall immune health.

6. Improved Sleep Quality

Better Sleep Patterns: Engaging in regular physical activity helps regulate sleep patterns by promoting deeper and more restorative sleep. Exercise can improve sleep quality and reduce symptoms of insomnia and other sleep disorders.

Increased Energy Levels: By enhancing overall physical fitness, exercise increases energy levels and reduces feelings of fatigue. This contributes to better daily functioning and improved overall quality of life.

7. Social Benefits

Opportunities for Social Interaction: Participating in group exercises or sports provides opportunities for social interaction and community building. Engaging in physical activities with others can foster relationships and provide a sense of belonging.

Enhanced Motivation and Accountability: Exercising with a partner or in a group can increase motivation and adherence to a fitness routine. The social aspect of group exercise can make workouts more enjoyable and help individuals stay committed to their fitness goals.

8. Long-Term Health Benefits

Increased Longevity: Regular physical activity is associated with a longer lifespan. Studies have shown that individuals who engage in regular exercise have a reduced risk of premature death and age-related diseases.

Improved Quality of Life: Exercise contributes to a higher quality of life by enhancing physical, mental, and emotional health. It supports independence and functional ability as individuals age, leading to a more active and fulfilling life.

Incorporating regular physical exercise into your daily routine offers a multitude of benefits that extend beyond physical health. From improving cardiovascular function and managing weight to enhancing mental well-being and fostering social connections, exercise is a powerful tool for achieving and maintaining overall health. By making physical activity a consistent part of your lifestyle, you can enjoy a range of positive outcomes that contribute to a longer, healthier, and more vibrant life.

Choosing the Right Type of Exercise for Your Body

Selecting the right type of exercise is crucial for achieving optimal health and fitness while minimizing the risk of injury and ensuring long-term adherence to a physical activity routine. Different types of exercise offer unique benefits, and finding the right fit for your body, fitness level, and personal preferences can significantly impact your overall well-being. Here's a guide to help you choose the most suitable exercise types based on various factors.

1. Assess Your Fitness Goals

Weight Loss: If your primary goal is weight loss, focus on exercises that increase calorie expenditure and boost metabolism. Cardiovascular exercises such as running, cycling, and swimming are effective for burning calories. High-intensity interval training (HIIT) can also be beneficial due to its ability to elevate the metabolic rate even after the workout.

Muscle Building: For muscle building, strength training exercises are essential. Incorporate resistance exercises like weight lifting, bodyweight exercises (push-ups, squats), and resistance band workouts. Target different muscle groups with various exercises to ensure balanced muscle development.

Cardiovascular Health: To improve cardiovascular health, engage in aerobic exercises that elevate your heart rate and enhance endurance. Activities such as brisk walking, jogging, dancing, and rowing are excellent choices for cardiovascular conditioning.

Flexibility and Mobility: If your goal is to enhance flexibility and mobility, incorporate stretching exercises and activities like yoga or Pilates. These practices improve range of motion, reduce stiffness, and support overall joint health.

Stress Relief: For managing stress and improving mental well-being, consider exercises that promote relaxation and mindfulness. Yoga, Tai Chi, and meditation-focused activities can help reduce stress and foster a sense of calm.

2. Consider Your Fitness Level

Beginner: If you're new to exercise, start with low-impact activities to build endurance and strength gradually. Walking, swimming, and cycling are gentle on the joints and suitable for beginners. As you progress, you can incorporate more challenging exercises like bodyweight workouts and light resistance training.

Intermediate: For those with some experience in fitness, a combination of moderate-intensity cardio and strength training exercises can be effective. Incorporate a mix of activities, such as running combined with weight lifting, to enhance overall fitness and prevent workout monotony.

Advanced: Experienced individuals may benefit from a diverse and advanced exercise routine that includes high-intensity interval training (HIIT), advanced resistance training, and complex functional movements. Tailor your routine to include exercises that challenge your strength, speed, and endurance.

3. Account for Personal Preferences

Enjoyment: Choose exercises that you enjoy to ensure adherence and long-term commitment. Whether it's dancing, hiking, or playing a sport, engaging in activities that bring you joy will make it easier to maintain a consistent workout routine.

Variety: Incorporate a variety of exercises to prevent boredom and keep your routine exciting. Combining different types of workouts, such as cardio, strength training, and flexibility exercises, can provide comprehensive fitness benefits and prevent plateauing.

Social Aspects: If you enjoy social interaction, consider group exercises or team sports. Group fitness classes, such as spin, aerobics, or martial arts, offer a social environment and can boost motivation through camaraderie.

4. Consider Any Physical Limitations

Injuries or Chronic Conditions: If you have a history of injuries or chronic conditions, choose low-impact exercises that minimize stress on the affected areas. Swimming, water aerobics, and cycling are excellent options for those with joint issues or orthopedic concerns.

Age and Mobility: For older adults or individuals with mobility limitations, focus on exercises that improve balance, coordination, and overall functionality. Activities like chair exercises, gentle stretching, and walking can be adapted to suit individual needs and capabilities.

5. Designing a Balanced Routine

Cardio: Incorporate cardiovascular exercises to improve heart health and endurance. Aim for at least 150 minutes of moderate-intensity cardio or 75 minutes of vigorous-intensity cardio per week.

Strength Training: Include strength training exercises to build muscle and support bone health. Aim for at least two sessions per week, targeting major muscle groups with exercises such as weight lifting, bodyweight movements, or resistance band workouts.

Flexibility: Add flexibility exercises to improve range of motion and prevent injuries. Incorporate stretching or yoga sessions 2-3 times per week to maintain flexibility and joint health.

Recovery: Allow for adequate recovery time between workouts to prevent overtraining and promote muscle repair. Incorporate rest days into your routine and consider active recovery activities like gentle stretching or light walking.

6. Seeking Professional Guidance

Personal Trainer: If you're unsure about designing an appropriate exercise routine, consider working with a certified personal trainer. A trainer can help assess your fitness level, set goals, and create a customized workout plan tailored to your needs.

Fitness Assessment: Conducting a fitness assessment with a healthcare provider or fitness professional can help identify your current fitness level, strengths, and areas for improvement. This information can guide you in selecting the most effective exercises for your goals.

Choosing the right type of exercise involves assessing your fitness goals, considering your fitness level and personal preferences, and accounting for any physical limitations. By designing a balanced routine that includes cardiovascular, strength, flexibility, and recovery components, you can achieve comprehensive health benefits and maintain long-term adherence to your fitness regimen. Whether you prefer solo workouts, group classes, or sports, finding activities that you enjoy and that suit your individual needs will support your overall well-being and fitness journey.

Integrating Movement into a Busy Lifestyle

Incorporating regular physical activity into a busy schedule can be challenging but is crucial for maintaining overall health and well-being. Finding creative and efficient ways to integrate movement into your daily life ensures that you stay active even when time is limited. Here's a comprehensive guide to seamlessly integrating movement into a busy lifestyle:

1. Prioritize Movement as Part of Your Routine

Making physical activity a priority helps to ensure it becomes a consistent part of your daily routine.

- **Schedule Workouts:** Treat your exercise time as an important appointment. Schedule specific times for physical activity in your calendar, just like you would for meetings or deadlines.

- **Create a Routine:** Develop a structured exercise routine that fits your schedule. Consistency is key, so choose times that work best for you and stick to them.

2. Incorporate Movement into Daily Tasks

Find ways to add physical activity to your existing daily tasks and routines.

- **Take the Stairs:** Opt for stairs instead of elevators or escalators whenever possible. This simple change can add extra steps to your day.

- **Walk or Bike to Work:** If feasible, walk or bike to work instead of driving. Alternatively, park farther away from your destination to increase your daily step count.

- **Stand and Move:** Use a standing desk or take regular breaks to stand up and stretch or walk around if you work at a desk. Incorporate mini-movements like calf raises or seated leg lifts.

3. Use Short, High-Intensity Workouts

Short, high-intensity workouts can be effective and efficient for busy schedules.

- **High-Intensity Interval Training (HIIT):** Engage in HIIT workouts, which involve short bursts of intense exercise followed by brief rest periods. HIIT can be completed in 20-30 minutes and provides a significant fitness boost.

- **Circuit Training:** Perform a series of exercises with minimal rest between each. Circuit training can be completed quickly and targets multiple muscle groups.

4. Incorporate Movement into Social Activities

Combine social interactions with physical activity to stay engaged and active.

- **Active Outings:** Plan active outings with friends or family, such as hiking, biking, or playing sports. Social activities that involve movement can be enjoyable and provide an opportunity to stay fit.

- **Group Classes:** Join fitness classes or group activities that fit your schedule. Group classes can provide motivation and accountability while fitting into your social life.

5. Utilize Technology and Apps

Leverage technology to help you stay on track with your movement goals.

- **Fitness Apps:** Use fitness apps to track your activity, set goals, and receive workout suggestions. Many apps offer short, effective workouts that can be done at home or during breaks.

- **Wearable Devices:** Invest in a fitness tracker or smartwatch to monitor your daily steps, heart rate, and overall activity levels. These devices can help keep you motivated and accountable.

6. Break Up Long Periods of Inactivity

Find ways to break up long periods of sitting or inactivity throughout your day.

- **Set Reminders:** Use reminders or alarms to prompt you to stand up, stretch, or walk around every 30-60 minutes. This can help counteract the negative effects of prolonged sitting.

- **Active Breaks:** Incorporate quick exercise routines into your breaks, such as stretching, bodyweight exercises, or a brisk walk.

7. Opt for Functional Exercises

Choose exercises that integrate movement into daily activities and functional tasks.

- **Functional Movements:** Engage in exercises that mimic everyday activities, such as squats, lunges, and kettlebell swings. These functional movements improve strength and flexibility for daily tasks.

- **Active Commuting:** Combine commuting with physical activity by walking or cycling to work, or use public transportation with added walking time.

8. Involve Family and Friends

Encourage family members or friends to join you in physical activities, making it a shared experience.

- **Family Activities:** Plan family outings that include physical activity, such as playing outdoor games, going for walks, or participating in recreational sports.
- **Workout Buddies:** Find a workout buddy to join you in exercise sessions. Exercising with someone can make the experience more enjoyable and provide mutual support.

9. Make the Most of Small Opportunities

Seize every opportunity to add movement into your day, even in small ways.

- **Active Household Chores:** Use household chores as a way to stay active. Activities such as cleaning, gardening, and DIY projects involve physical movement.
- **Mini-Workouts:** Perform quick, bodyweight exercises during short breaks or while waiting for appointments. Examples include jumping jacks, planks, or high knees.

10. Emphasize Enjoyment and Variety

Choose activities that you enjoy and that fit your preferences to stay motivated and engaged.

- **Explore Different Activities:** Try various forms of exercise to find what you enjoy most, whether it's dancing, swimming, yoga, or martial arts.
- **Mix It Up:** Keep your routine interesting by varying your workouts. Incorporate different activities and routines to prevent boredom and maintain enthusiasm.

Integrating movement into a busy lifestyle involves prioritizing physical activity, incorporating it into daily tasks, utilizing short and effective workouts, and leveraging technology. By making movement a natural and enjoyable part of your routine, you can maintain a healthy and active lifestyle despite a hectic schedule. Remember, even small changes can have a significant impact on your overall well-being, and finding ways to stay active every day will contribute to your long-term health and vitality.

Chapter 6: I - Immune Support

Strengthening Your Immune System Naturally

A strong immune system is essential for protecting your body against infections, diseases, and various health challenges. While conventional medicine and vaccines play a crucial role in maintaining health, there are also natural ways to support and enhance your immune system. Here's how you can strengthen your immune system through lifestyle changes, nutrition, and natural remedies:

1. Adopt a Balanced Diet

Nutrient-Rich Foods: Incorporate a variety of nutrient-dense foods into your diet to support immune function. Focus on fruits, vegetables, whole grains, nuts, and seeds. These foods provide essential vitamins, minerals, and antioxidants that help maintain immune health.

Key Nutrients:

- **Vitamin C:** Found in citrus fruits, bell peppers, strawberries, and broccoli. Vitamin C is known for its immune-boosting properties and its role in collagen production.

- **Vitamin D:** Essential for immune function and can be obtained from sunlight, fatty fish (like salmon), fortified dairy products, and supplements.

- **Zinc:** Found in nuts, seeds, legumes, and whole grains. Zinc is crucial for immune cell function and wound healing.

- **Omega-3 Fatty Acids:** Present in fatty fish, flaxseeds, and walnuts. Omega-3s have anti-inflammatory properties and support overall immune health.

Hydration: Stay well-hydrated by drinking plenty of water throughout the day. Proper hydration supports the health of every cell in your body, including those involved in immune responses.

2. Maintain a Healthy Weight

Balanced Diet and Exercise: Achieving and maintaining a healthy weight through a balanced diet and regular physical activity can enhance immune function. Obesity can impair immune response, making it more challenging for the body to fight infections.

Healthy Eating Habits: Avoid excessive consumption of processed foods, sugary snacks, and unhealthy fats. Instead, focus on whole foods that provide essential nutrients and support overall health.

3. Regular Physical Activity

Exercise Benefits: Engage in regular physical activity to strengthen your immune system. Exercise promotes good circulation, which helps immune cells move throughout the body and perform their functions effectively.

Types of Exercise:

- **Aerobic Exercise:** Activities like walking, jogging, and cycling improve cardiovascular health and boost immune function.

- **Strength Training:** Incorporate resistance exercises to support muscle health and overall fitness.

- **Moderation:** Aim for at least 150 minutes of moderate-intensity exercise or 75 minutes of vigorous exercise per week, combined with muscle-strengthening activities on two or more days.

4. Prioritize Quality Sleep

Sleep and Immunity: Adequate and restful sleep is vital for a healthy immune system. During sleep, the body produces cytokines and other immune factors that help combat infections and inflammation.

Healthy Sleep Habits:

- **Establish a Routine:** Go to bed and wake up at the same time every day, even on weekends.

- **Create a Sleep-Friendly Environment:** Ensure your bedroom is dark, quiet, and cool. Invest in a comfortable mattress and pillow.

- **Limit Stimulants:** Avoid caffeine, alcohol, and electronic screens before bedtime.

5. Manage Stress Effectively

Impact of Stress: Chronic stress can suppress immune function and increase susceptibility to illnesses. Effective stress management techniques can help maintain a strong immune system.

Stress Reduction Strategies:

- **Mindfulness and Meditation:** Practice mindfulness techniques and meditation to reduce stress and promote relaxation.

- **Deep Breathing Exercises:** Engage in deep breathing exercises to calm the nervous system and reduce stress levels.

- **Relaxation Techniques:** Activities such as yoga, Tai Chi, and progressive muscle relaxation can help alleviate stress and support immune health.

6. Support Digestive Health

Gut Health and Immunity: A healthy gut microbiome is essential for a well-functioning immune system. The gut microbiome plays a crucial role in modulating immune responses and protecting against pathogens.

Probiotics and Prebiotics:

- **Probiotics:** Consume probiotic-rich foods like yogurt, kefir, sauerkraut, and kimchi to promote beneficial gut bacteria.

- **Prebiotics:** Include prebiotic foods like garlic, onions, bananas, and asparagus to support the growth of healthy gut flora.

Fiber Intake: A diet high in dietary fiber supports gut health and immune function. Aim to include a variety of fiber-rich foods such as fruits, vegetables, legumes, and whole grains.

7. Incorporate Immune-Boosting Herbs and Supplements

Herbal Remedies:

- **Echinacea:** Known for its immune-stimulating properties, Echinacea may help reduce the duration and severity of colds.

- **Elderberry:** Elderberry extracts have been shown to have antiviral properties and may help alleviate flu symptoms.

- **Garlic:** Garlic has antimicrobial and immune-boosting properties that can support overall health.

Supplements:

- **Vitamin C:** Consider supplements if you're not getting enough from your diet, especially during cold and flu season.

- **Vitamin D:** Supplementation may be necessary, particularly in areas with limited sunlight exposure.

- **Probiotics:** Supplement with probiotics to support gut health and immune function.

8. Avoid Harmful Habits

Limit Alcohol Consumption: Excessive alcohol intake can weaken the immune system and impair the body's ability to fight infections. Limit alcohol consumption to moderate levels.

Quit Smoking: Smoking damages the respiratory system and impairs immune function. Quitting smoking improves overall health and enhances immune response.

Strengthening your immune system naturally involves a holistic approach that includes a balanced diet, regular physical activity, quality sleep, stress management, and support for digestive health. By adopting these strategies and incorporating immune-boosting herbs and supplements, you can enhance your body's ability to defend against illnesses and promote long-term well-being. Prioritizing these practices in your daily life will contribute to a stronger, more resilient immune system.

The Role of Nutrition, Sleep, and Stress Management in Immunity

A well-functioning immune system is crucial for defending the body against pathogens and maintaining overall health. Three key factors—nutrition, sleep, and stress management—play significant roles in supporting and enhancing immune function. Understanding how these elements interact can help you adopt a holistic approach to strengthen your immune system.

1. Nutrition and Immunity

Essential Nutrients: Proper nutrition provides the building blocks for a strong immune system. Certain nutrients are particularly important for immune health:

- **Vitamin C:** Found in citrus fruits, strawberries, bell peppers, and broccoli, Vitamin C supports the production of white blood cells and enhances the function of immune cells. It also acts as an antioxidant, protecting cells from damage.

- **Vitamin D:** Obtained from sunlight, fatty fish, and fortified foods, Vitamin D regulates immune responses and helps activate immune cells. Low levels of Vitamin D have been linked to increased susceptibility to infections.

- **Zinc:** Present in nuts, seeds, legumes, and whole grains, zinc is crucial for the development and function of immune cells. It also helps in wound healing and DNA synthesis.

- **Omega-3 Fatty Acids:** Found in fatty fish, flaxseeds, and walnuts, omega-3s have anti-inflammatory properties and support overall immune function.

Balanced Diet: A well-rounded diet that includes a variety of fruits, vegetables, whole grains, lean proteins, and healthy fats ensures that you get the necessary nutrients to support immune health. Avoid excessive consumption of processed foods, sugary snacks, and unhealthy fats, which can negatively impact immune function.

Hydration: Adequate hydration is vital for maintaining the health of every cell in your body, including those involved in immune responses. Drink plenty of water throughout the day to support overall health and immune function.

2. Sleep and Immunity

Importance of Sleep: Quality sleep is essential for a robust immune system. During sleep, the body produces and releases cytokines and other immune factors that help fight infections and inflammation. Poor sleep can impair immune function and increase susceptibility to illnesses.

Sleep Stages:

- **Deep Sleep:** This stage is crucial for physical restoration and immune system maintenance. It allows for the production of immune cells and proteins that are essential for fighting infections.

- **REM Sleep:** REM sleep is important for cognitive function and emotional health, which indirectly supports immune health by reducing stress and promoting overall well-being.

Healthy Sleep Habits:

- **Consistency:** Go to bed and wake up at the same time each day to regulate your sleep-wake cycle.

- **Sleep Environment:** Ensure your bedroom is conducive to sleep by keeping it dark, quiet, and cool.

- **Pre-Sleep Routine:** Avoid stimulants such as caffeine and electronic screens before bedtime. Establish a relaxing pre-sleep routine to prepare your body for rest.

3. Stress Management and Immunity

Impact of Stress: Chronic stress can weaken the immune system by affecting the production and function of immune cells. Stress activates the body's "fight or flight" response, leading to the release of stress hormones like cortisol, which can suppress immune function and increase vulnerability to infections.

Stress Response:

- **Acute Stress:** Short-term stress can mobilize the immune system, providing a temporary boost in immune response. However, chronic stress can lead to prolonged immune suppression.

- **Chronic Stress:** Persistent stress can result in ongoing inflammation and immune dysregulation, increasing the risk of chronic diseases and infections.

Stress Management Techniques:

- **Mindfulness and Meditation:** Practicing mindfulness and meditation can help calm the nervous system and reduce stress levels. Techniques such as deep breathing, progressive muscle relaxation, and guided imagery are effective for managing stress.

- **Physical Activity:** Regular exercise is a powerful stress reliever and has been shown to improve mood and immune function. Aim for at least 150 minutes of moderate-intensity exercise per week.

- **Healthy Lifestyle Choices:** Maintaining a balanced diet, staying hydrated, and getting sufficient sleep contribute to overall stress reduction and support immune health.

Social Support: Building and maintaining positive relationships and social connections can help manage stress and enhance emotional well-being. Support from friends and family provides emotional comfort and practical assistance, reducing the impact of stress on your immune system.

Nutrition, sleep, and stress management are integral components of a healthy immune system. By adopting a balanced diet rich in essential nutrients, prioritizing quality sleep, and effectively managing stress, you can support and enhance your immune function. These holistic practices not only strengthen your body's defenses but also contribute to overall well-being and resilience. Embracing these elements as part of your daily routine will help maintain a robust immune system and promote long-term health.

Herbal Remedies and Supplements for Immune Health

In addition to a balanced diet and a healthy lifestyle, herbal remedies and supplements can play a significant role in supporting and enhancing immune health. Various herbs and supplements have been studied for their potential to bolster the immune system, reduce inflammation, and aid in the prevention of illnesses. Here's a comprehensive overview of some of the most effective herbal remedies and supplements for immune support:

1. Herbal Remedies

Echinacea:

- **Benefits:** Echinacea is widely used to prevent and treat the common cold. It is believed to stimulate the production of white blood cells and enhance immune function.
- **Forms:** Available as teas, tinctures, capsules, and extracts.
- **Usage:** Take Echinacea at the onset of cold symptoms or during flu season. Dosage may vary based on the form and concentration.

Elderberry:

- **Benefits:** Elderberry is known for its antiviral properties and is often used to alleviate flu symptoms. It contains compounds that may inhibit viral replication and reduce inflammation.
- **Forms:** Available as syrups, lozenges, and capsules.
- **Usage:** Begin using elderberry at the first sign of flu symptoms for potential relief.

Garlic:

- **Benefits:** Garlic has antimicrobial and immune-boosting properties. It can enhance the immune system's ability to fight off infections and has been shown to have anti-inflammatory effects.
- **Forms:** Fresh garlic, garlic supplements, or garlic-infused oils.

- **Usage:** Incorporate garlic into your diet regularly or take supplements as directed.

Ginger:

- **Benefits:** Ginger is known for its anti-inflammatory and antioxidant properties. It can help soothe the throat, support digestion, and strengthen the immune system.
- **Forms:** Fresh ginger, ginger tea, capsules, or powdered ginger.
- **Usage:** Drink ginger tea or add fresh ginger to meals for regular immune support.

Turmeric:

- **Benefits:** Turmeric contains curcumin, a compound with strong anti-inflammatory and antioxidant properties. It can help modulate immune responses and reduce inflammation.
- **Forms:** Turmeric powder, capsules, or extracts.
- **Usage:** Use turmeric as a spice in cooking or take supplements according to recommended dosages.

Astragalus:

- **Benefits:** Astragalus is an adaptogenic herb that can help support the immune system and enhance the body's resistance to stress.
- **Forms:** Capsules, tinctures, or teas.
- **Usage:** Use Astragalus regularly to support long-term immune health.

2. Supplements for Immune Health

Vitamin C:

- **Benefits:** Vitamin C is a powerful antioxidant that supports the production and function of immune cells. It can help reduce the severity and duration of colds.
- **Forms:** Available as tablets, capsules, powders, and gummies.
- **Usage:** Take Vitamin C daily, especially during cold and flu season. The recommended dosage may vary based on individual needs.

Vitamin D:

- **Benefits:** Vitamin D plays a crucial role in regulating immune responses and enhancing the function of immune cells. Deficiency in Vitamin D has been linked to increased susceptibility to infections.

- **Forms:** Available as tablets, capsules, drops, and gummies.

- **Usage:** Take Vitamin D supplements, particularly in areas with limited sunlight exposure, or as advised by a healthcare professional.

Zinc:

- **Benefits:** Zinc is essential for immune cell development and function. It can help reduce the duration of cold symptoms and support overall immune health.

- **Forms:** Available as tablets, lozenges, and capsules.

- **Usage:** Take Zinc supplements as directed, especially during cold season or if you have a deficiency.

Probiotics:

- **Benefits:** Probiotics support gut health, which is closely linked to immune function. A healthy gut microbiome helps regulate immune responses and protect against pathogens.

- **Forms:** Available as capsules, tablets, powders, and fermented foods.

- **Usage:** Incorporate probiotic supplements or probiotic-rich foods into your diet regularly.

Elderberry Extract:

- **Benefits:** Similar to elderberry itself, elderberry extract can help support immune function and alleviate cold and flu symptoms.

- **Forms:** Available as liquid extracts, capsules, and gummies.

- **Usage:** Use elderberry extract according to the manufacturer's recommendations, especially during flu season.

Beta-Glucans:

- **Benefits:** Beta-glucans are natural compounds found in oats, barley, and certain mushrooms. They can enhance immune response by activating immune cells.

- **Forms:** Available as supplements or in foods.

- **Usage:** Take beta-glucan supplements or include beta-glucan-rich foods in your diet.

3. Safety and Considerations

Consultation with Healthcare Providers: Before starting any new herbal remedy or supplement, consult with a healthcare provider, especially if you have underlying health conditions or are taking other medications. Some herbs and supplements can interact with medications or have side effects.

Quality and Dosage: Choose high-quality products from reputable manufacturers. Follow recommended dosages and usage instructions to avoid potential adverse effects.

Balanced Approach: While herbal remedies and supplements can support immune health, they should be used as part of a comprehensive approach that includes a balanced diet, regular exercise, quality sleep, and effective stress management.

Herbal remedies and supplements can be valuable tools in supporting and enhancing immune health. By incorporating these natural options into a balanced lifestyle, you can help strengthen your body's defenses and promote overall well-being. Always consult with a healthcare provider to ensure that the remedies and supplements you choose are appropriate for your individual health needs.

Chapter 7: N - Nourish

Understanding the Concept of Nourishment Beyond Food

Nourishment is often thought of in terms of food and nutrients, but true well-being extends beyond what we eat. The concept of nourishment encompasses a broader range of factors that contribute to holistic health and vitality. Understanding nourishment in its entirety involves recognizing the various ways we can support our physical, emotional, and spiritual well-being. Here's a detailed exploration of nourishment beyond food:

1. Emotional Nourishment

Emotional Well-Being: Emotional nourishment involves addressing and nurturing our emotional needs. It includes cultivating a positive self-image, managing stress, and maintaining emotional resilience. Emotional well-being is crucial for overall health and can influence how we experience and respond to life's challenges.

Supportive Relationships: Building and maintaining strong, supportive relationships with family, friends, and communities provide emotional nourishment. Positive social connections offer a sense of belonging, support during difficult times, and opportunities for joy and shared experiences.

Self-Care Practices: Engaging in activities that promote relaxation and self-care is essential for emotional health. This can include hobbies, leisure activities, and time spent on activities that bring joy and fulfillment.

Therapeutic Support: Seeking support from mental health professionals when needed can also be a form of emotional nourishment. Therapy and counseling provide tools and strategies for managing emotional difficulties and improving mental well-being.

2. Spiritual Nourishment

Purpose and Meaning: Spiritual nourishment involves finding purpose and meaning in life. This can be achieved through personal values, beliefs, and practices that align with one's sense of purpose. Exploring and nurturing spiritual beliefs can offer a deeper sense of connection and fulfillment.

Mindfulness and Meditation: Practices such as mindfulness and meditation help connect with one's inner self and promote spiritual growth. These practices foster a sense of peace, clarity, and connection to something greater than oneself.

Community and Belonging: Participating in spiritual or religious communities can provide a sense of belonging and support. Shared values and communal activities contribute to a sense of connection and provide opportunities for spiritual growth and reflection.

Reflection and Gratitude: Incorporating practices of reflection and gratitude into daily life helps foster a sense of appreciation and awareness. Keeping a gratitude journal or engaging in reflective practices can enhance spiritual well-being and overall satisfaction.

3. Intellectual Nourishment

Continuous Learning: Intellectual nourishment involves stimulating the mind and engaging in continuous learning. This can include reading, pursuing education, or exploring new interests and hobbies. Keeping the mind active and curious promotes cognitive health and personal growth.

Critical Thinking: Engaging in activities that challenge your thinking and encourage critical analysis helps maintain cognitive function. Discussions, debates, and problem-solving activities stimulate intellectual engagement and growth.

Creative Expression: Participating in creative activities such as writing, art, music, or other forms of self-expression nourishes the intellect and provides an outlet for personal creativity and innovation.

4. Physical Nourishment

Movement and Exercise: Physical nourishment goes beyond nutrition to include regular physical activity. Exercise supports overall health by improving cardiovascular function, boosting mood, and enhancing energy levels. Incorporating movement into daily life is essential for maintaining physical vitality.

Rest and Recovery: Adequate rest and recovery are vital components of physical nourishment. This includes not only sufficient sleep but also allowing time for relaxation and recovery after physical exertion.

Environmental Factors: Creating a healthy living environment, such as maintaining clean air and water, and ensuring a safe and comfortable living space, contributes to overall physical well-being. The environment in which we live can significantly impact our health and quality of life.

5. Social Nourishment

Community Engagement: Being involved in social and community activities provides a sense of connection and support. Engaging with others through social groups, volunteer work, and community events fosters a sense of belonging and enriches life experiences.

Healthy Relationships: Building and maintaining healthy, positive relationships is a key aspect of social nourishment. Relationships characterized by mutual respect, support, and communication contribute to overall well-being and happiness.

Social Support Networks: Having access to a supportive social network helps in managing life's challenges and enhances emotional resilience. Social support provides practical assistance, emotional comfort, and a sense of connection during difficult times.

Nourishment extends far beyond the food we consume. It encompasses emotional, spiritual, intellectual, physical, and social dimensions of well-being. By recognizing and nurturing these various aspects, we can achieve a more balanced and fulfilling life. Embracing a holistic approach to nourishment allows for a deeper sense of health and vitality, supporting not just physical wellness but also emotional and spiritual richness.

The Role of Emotional and Spiritual Health in Physical Well-Being

Emotional and spiritual health are deeply interconnected with physical well-being, influencing not only how we feel mentally and emotionally but also how our bodies function and respond to various health challenges. Understanding this connection highlights the importance of addressing emotional and spiritual needs as integral components of overall health.

1. Emotional Health and Physical Well-Being

Stress and Physical Health:

- **Impact:** Chronic stress can lead to a range of physical health issues, including cardiovascular problems, gastrointestinal disorders, and weakened immune function. The body's stress response involves the release of hormones such as cortisol and adrenaline, which, when persistently elevated, can contribute to inflammation and other health problems.

- **Management:** Effective stress management techniques, such as mindfulness, relaxation exercises, and therapy, can help mitigate the physical effects of stress and promote better health outcomes.

Emotional Resilience:

- **Impact:** Emotional resilience—the ability to bounce back from adversity—can positively influence physical health. Individuals with high emotional resilience are better equipped to handle stress and recover from illness more quickly.

- **Support:** Building emotional resilience through support networks, therapy, and positive coping strategies can enhance physical health by reducing the impact of stress and improving overall well-being.

Mood and Immune Function:

- **Impact:** Emotional states such as depression and anxiety can impair immune function, making individuals more susceptible to infections and illnesses. Positive emotions and a sense of well-being, on the other hand, can boost immune responses and improve health outcomes.

- **Enhancement:** Engaging in activities that promote positive emotions, such as social interactions, hobbies, and self-care, can support immune health and contribute to overall physical well-being.

2. Spiritual Health and Physical Well-Being

Purpose and Meaning:

- **Impact:** A sense of purpose and meaning in life can positively influence physical health by providing motivation and reducing stress. Individuals who feel that their lives have meaning are often more resilient in the face of illness and are better able to cope with health challenges.

- **Cultivation:** Finding and nurturing a sense of purpose through personal values, goals, and spiritual practices can enhance overall well-being and support physical health.

Mind-Body Connection:

- **Impact:** Spiritual practices such as meditation and prayer can influence the body's physiological processes. These practices often lead to reduced stress, lower blood pressure, and improved overall health by fostering relaxation and enhancing emotional balance.

- **Practice:** Incorporating mindfulness, meditation, or spiritual rituals into daily life can support physical health by promoting relaxation and reducing the physiological impact of stress.

Community and Support:

- **Impact:** Being part of a spiritual or religious community provides social support, which can positively affect physical health. Social support helps reduce stress, fosters a sense of belonging, and provides resources for managing health issues.

- **Engagement:** Participation in community or spiritual groups can offer emotional support and practical assistance, contributing to improved physical health and overall well-being.

3. Integration of Emotional and Spiritual Health

Holistic Approach:

- **Impact:** Addressing both emotional and spiritual health as part of a holistic approach to well-being recognizes the interconnectedness of mind, body, and spirit. Integrating practices that support emotional balance and spiritual growth can enhance physical health outcomes.

- **Implementation:** Developing a balanced approach that includes emotional support, stress management, spiritual practices, and physical health care can lead to a more comprehensive and effective health strategy.

Self-Care and Balance:

- **Impact:** Prioritizing self-care and maintaining balance between emotional, spiritual, and physical health is essential for overall well-being. Neglecting one aspect can negatively affect others, leading to imbalances and health issues.

- **Strategy:** Create a self-care plan that includes emotional and spiritual practices alongside physical health activities. This balanced approach helps maintain harmony and supports overall health.

Emotional and spiritual health play a crucial role in physical well-being, influencing how the body responds to stress, illness, and overall health challenges. By recognizing and addressing the interconnectedness of emotional, spiritual, and physical health, individuals can achieve a more holistic and effective approach to well-being. Cultivating emotional resilience, finding purpose and meaning, and engaging in supportive practices contribute to enhanced physical health and a richer, more fulfilling life.

Building Resilience Through Positive Relationships and Community

Resilience is the ability to adapt and recover from adversity, stress, and challenges. One of the most powerful factors in building and maintaining resilience is the presence of positive relationships and supportive communities. These social connections play a critical role in enhancing emotional strength, providing support during tough times, and fostering overall well-being. Here's an in-depth exploration of how positive relationships and community contribute to resilience:

1. The Power of Positive Relationships

Emotional Support:

- **Impact:** Positive relationships provide a crucial source of emotional support. Friends, family members, and loved ones offer empathy, understanding, and reassurance, helping individuals navigate stress and challenges with greater ease.

- **Mechanism:** Emotional support can buffer against the negative effects of stress, reduce feelings of isolation, and provide comfort during difficult times.

Encouragement and Motivation:

- **Impact:** Supportive relationships encourage and motivate individuals to pursue their goals, overcome obstacles, and maintain a positive outlook. Encouragement from others can boost self-confidence and persistence.

- **Mechanism:** Positive reinforcement and constructive feedback from loved ones help individuals stay motivated and committed to their personal and professional aspirations.

Stress Relief:

- **Impact:** Engaging with supportive people can reduce stress levels and promote relaxation. Social interactions often provide a break from stressors and offer a chance to unwind and enjoy moments of joy.

- **Mechanism:** Sharing experiences, discussing concerns, and receiving validation from others help alleviate feelings of stress and promote emotional well-being.

2. The Role of Community in Building Resilience

Sense of Belonging:

- **Impact:** Being part of a community provides a sense of belonging and connection. This sense of inclusion and acceptance helps individuals feel valued and supported, which can enhance resilience.

- **Mechanism:** Community involvement fosters social bonds and shared experiences, contributing to a strong support network that individuals can rely on during challenging times.

Collective Support:

- **Impact:** Communities often offer collective resources and support systems that individuals can access. This includes practical assistance, such as access to services and resources, as well as emotional and social support.

- **Mechanism:** Community resources, such as support groups, volunteer organizations, and social services, provide practical help and emotional support, enhancing resilience.

Shared Experiences:

- **Impact:** Sharing experiences with others who have faced similar challenges can provide comfort and insights. This shared understanding fosters empathy and offers practical strategies for coping and overcoming difficulties.

- **Mechanism:** Peer support and community connections allow individuals to learn from others' experiences and gain perspective, which can be empowering and reassuring.

3. Cultivating and Maintaining Positive Relationships

Building Trust:

- **Approach:** Establishing and maintaining trust is essential for positive relationships. Open communication, honesty, and reliability strengthen trust and deepen connections.

- **Practice:** Actively listening, being supportive, and respecting others' boundaries contribute to building and sustaining trust in relationships.

Fostering Communication:

- **Approach:** Effective communication is key to healthy relationships. Clear, empathetic, and respectful communication helps prevent misunderstandings and resolve conflicts constructively.

- **Practice:** Engage in regular, meaningful conversations, express feelings and concerns openly, and practice active listening.

Nurturing Connections:

- **Approach:** Invest time and effort in nurturing relationships. Regular interactions, shared activities, and expressing appreciation help maintain and strengthen bonds.

- **Practice:** Spend quality time with loved ones, participate in activities together, and show gratitude and affection.

4. Engaging with the Community

Participation:

- **Approach:** Actively participate in community activities and organizations to build connections and contribute to collective well-being. Engagement fosters a sense of belonging and provides opportunities for social support.

- **Practice:** Volunteer for local events, join community groups or clubs, and participate in social and civic activities.

Building Networks:

- **Approach:** Expand and strengthen social networks by connecting with diverse individuals and groups. Building a broad network of relationships provides additional sources of support and resources.

- **Practice:** Attend networking events, join interest-based groups, and engage in community forums and discussions.

Creating Supportive Environments:

- **Approach:** Contribute to creating a supportive and inclusive community environment. Advocate for positive change and support initiatives that promote collective well-being.

- **Practice:** Get involved in community advocacy, support local causes, and promote inclusivity and support within the community.

Positive relationships and community play a fundamental role in building and sustaining resilience. Emotional support, encouragement, and a sense of belonging enhance individual and collective well-being, providing a strong foundation for coping with adversity. By cultivating trust, effective communication, and active community engagement, individuals can strengthen their resilience and navigate life's challenges with greater confidence and support. Investing in positive relationships and community connections not only fosters personal resilience but also contributes to a more supportive and connected society.

Chapter 8: M – Mindset

The Power of Positive Thinking in Healing

Positive thinking is more than just an optimistic outlook; it plays a significant role in physical, emotional, and mental healing. Research has shown that cultivating a positive mindset can impact health outcomes, support recovery, and enhance overall well-being. Here's a detailed exploration of the power of positive thinking in healing:

1. Understanding Positive Thinking

Definition and Principles:

- **Positive Thinking:** Refers to focusing on the positive aspects of life, expecting favorable outcomes, and maintaining an optimistic perspective even in the face of challenges.

- **Principles:** Involves cognitive reframing, gratitude practices, and developing a mindset that seeks opportunities and solutions rather than dwelling on problems.

Psychological Impact:

- **Impact:** Positive thinking influences mental health by reducing stress, anxiety, and depression. It helps individuals cope with difficulties more effectively and promotes a sense of hope and control.

- **Mechanism:** Positive thoughts trigger the release of neurotransmitters such as dopamine and serotonin, which are associated with improved mood and reduced stress levels.

2. Positive Thinking and Physical Health

Immune System Enhancement:

- **Impact:** Optimistic individuals often have stronger immune responses. Positive thinking has been linked to lower levels of inflammation and a reduced risk of chronic diseases.

- **Mechanism:** Positive emotions and reduced stress levels can enhance the functioning of the immune system, making the body more effective at fighting off infections and illnesses.

Pain Management:

- **Impact:** Positive thinking can help manage pain and improve pain tolerance. Patients with a positive outlook often report lower levels of pain and discomfort.

- **Mechanism:** Positive thinking can alter the perception of pain by focusing on positive aspects of recovery and employing mental techniques such as visualization and relaxation.

Cardiovascular Health:

- **Impact:** Optimism and positive thinking contribute to better cardiovascular health. Studies show that positive individuals have a lower risk of heart disease and better outcomes after cardiac events.

- **Mechanism:** Positive thinking reduces stress, which in turn lowers blood pressure and decreases the risk of cardiovascular complications.

3. The Role of Positive Thinking in Mental and Emotional Healing

Coping with Stress:

- **Impact:** Positive thinking improves resilience and coping abilities during stressful situations. It helps individuals manage stress more effectively and reduces the likelihood of developing stress-related disorders.

- **Mechanism:** By focusing on positive outcomes and solutions, individuals can navigate stress with a clearer perspective and greater emotional stability.

Enhancing Recovery:

- **Impact:** A positive mindset can accelerate recovery from illness or surgery. Patients who maintain an optimistic outlook tend to recover more quickly and experience fewer complications.

- **Mechanism:** Positive thinking promotes a proactive attitude towards recovery, encouraging adherence to treatment plans and fostering a greater sense of agency in the healing process.

Building Emotional Resilience:

- **Impact:** Positive thinking strengthens emotional resilience, enabling individuals to bounce back from adversity with greater ease. It fosters a sense of hope and determination.

- **Mechanism:** By maintaining a positive outlook, individuals can develop coping strategies and resilience skills that help them overcome challenges and setbacks.

4. Techniques for Cultivating Positive Thinking

Cognitive Reframing:

- **Technique:** Cognitive reframing involves changing negative or unhelpful thoughts into positive or constructive ones. This technique helps individuals shift their perspective and focus on solutions rather than problems.

- **Practice:** Identify negative thoughts and consciously replace them with positive affirmations or constructive thoughts. For example, change "I can't handle this" to "I am capable of finding a solution."

Gratitude Practice:

- **Technique:** Practicing gratitude involves regularly reflecting on and appreciating positive aspects of life. This practice enhances overall mood and fosters a positive mindset.

- **Practice:** Keep a gratitude journal, noting things you are thankful for each day. Express appreciation for positive experiences and people in your life.

Visualization and Affirmations:

- **Technique:** Visualization involves imagining positive outcomes and scenarios, while affirmations are positive statements that reinforce self-belief and optimism.

- **Practice:** Use visualization techniques to imagine successful outcomes and positive experiences. Repeat affirmations such as "I am healthy and strong" to reinforce a positive mindset.

Mindfulness and Meditation:

- **Technique:** Mindfulness and meditation practices help cultivate a present-focused and positive outlook. They reduce stress and enhance emotional well-being by fostering awareness and acceptance.

- **Practice:** Incorporate mindfulness meditation into your daily routine. Focus on the present moment, practice deep breathing, and engage in guided meditations that promote positivity.

5. Integrating Positive Thinking into Daily Life

Healthy Lifestyle Choices:

- **Integration:** Combine positive thinking with healthy lifestyle choices to support overall well-being. Engage in regular physical activity, eat a balanced diet, and prioritize self-care.

- **Practice:** Maintain a routine that includes exercise, nutritious meals, and relaxation techniques to complement a positive mindset and enhance overall health.

Supportive Environment:

- **Integration:** Surround yourself with supportive and positive individuals who uplift and encourage you. Create an environment that fosters positivity and well-being.

- **Practice:** Build relationships with people who share your values and encourage a positive outlook. Engage in social activities that bring joy and support.

Continuous Improvement:

- **Integration:** Continuously work on developing and maintaining a positive mindset. Embrace opportunities for personal growth and self-improvement.

- **Practice:** Set goals for personal development, seek new experiences, and engage in activities that promote positivity and resilience.

The power of positive thinking in healing is profound and multifaceted. By fostering a positive mindset, individuals can enhance their physical health, manage stress, and support emotional and mental well-being. Techniques such as cognitive reframing, gratitude practice, and mindfulness contribute to cultivating a positive outlook and improving overall health outcomes. Integrating positive thinking into daily life, alongside healthy lifestyle choices and supportive relationships, can lead to a more resilient and fulfilling life. Embracing positivity as a central component of health supports not only healing but also a richer, more vibrant life.

Cultivating a Growth Mindset for Lifelong Wellness

A growth mindset, a concept developed by psychologist Carol Dweck, refers to the belief that abilities and intelligence can be developed through dedication, effort, and learning. Cultivating a growth mindset is essential for lifelong wellness as it empowers individuals to embrace challenges, learn from experiences, and continuously improve their physical, emotional, and mental health. Here's a detailed exploration of how cultivating a growth mindset contributes to lifelong wellness:

1. Understanding a Growth Mindset

Definition and Characteristics:

- **Growth Mindset:** The belief that skills and intelligence can be developed through effort, learning, and perseverance. Individuals with a growth mindset view challenges as opportunities for growth rather than obstacles.

- **Characteristics:** Embracing challenges, persisting through difficulties, learning from criticism, and being inspired by the success of others.

Comparison with a Fixed Mindset:

- **Fixed Mindset:** The belief that abilities and intelligence are static and unchangeable. Individuals with a fixed mindset may avoid challenges, give up easily, and feel threatened by others' success.

- **Impact:** A fixed mindset can limit personal development and hinder progress, while a growth mindset fosters resilience, adaptability, and continuous improvement.

2. The Role of a Growth Mindset in Physical Health

Embracing Healthy Habits:

- **Impact:** Individuals with a growth mindset are more likely to adopt and maintain healthy lifestyle habits. They view health-related challenges as opportunities to learn and improve.

- **Practice:** Approach dietary changes, exercise routines, and wellness goals with curiosity and a willingness to adapt. View setbacks as learning experiences rather than failures.

Overcoming Obstacles:

- **Impact:** A growth mindset helps individuals overcome physical health obstacles and setbacks. It encourages persistence and creative problem-solving in the face of challenges.

- **Practice:** When encountering difficulties in achieving fitness goals or managing health conditions, use a growth mindset to seek solutions and adapt strategies.

Enhancing Resilience:

- **Impact:** Embracing a growth mindset enhances resilience and adaptability in managing physical health. It promotes a positive outlook and a proactive approach to health challenges.

- **Practice:** Develop resilience by focusing on incremental progress, learning from setbacks, and celebrating small victories in health and wellness.

3. The Impact of a Growth Mindset on Emotional Well-Being

Handling Stress and Adversity:

- **Impact:** A growth mindset helps individuals handle stress and adversity more effectively. It encourages viewing challenges as opportunities to develop coping skills and emotional strength.

- **Practice:** When faced with emotional stress, approach the situation with a growth mindset by exploring coping strategies, seeking support, and reflecting on personal growth.

Building Emotional Resilience:

- **Impact:** Individuals with a growth mindset build emotional resilience by embracing new experiences, learning from emotional challenges, and developing a positive attitude towards personal growth.

- **Practice:** Engage in activities that promote emotional growth, such as mindfulness, journaling, and seeking feedback from trusted sources.

Developing Positive Relationships:

- **Impact:** A growth mindset fosters healthy and positive relationships. It encourages open communication, empathy, and a willingness to learn and grow within relationships.

- **Practice:** Approach relationships with curiosity and a willingness to understand others' perspectives. Use conflicts and challenges as opportunities for growth and improved connection.

4. Applying a Growth Mindset to Mental Wellness

Continuous Learning and Self-Improvement:

- **Impact:** A growth mindset promotes continuous learning and self-improvement, contributing to mental wellness. It encourages individuals to seek out new knowledge, skills, and experiences.

- **Practice:** Pursue lifelong learning opportunities, set personal development goals, and seek feedback to enhance mental wellness and cognitive growth.

Embracing Change and Adaptability:

- **Impact:** A growth mindset enhances adaptability and openness to change, which is crucial for mental wellness. It helps individuals navigate transitions and challenges with resilience and optimism.

- **Practice:** Embrace change as an opportunity for growth, seek new experiences, and develop flexibility in adapting to life's evolving circumstances.

Managing Negative Thoughts:

- **Impact:** A growth mindset helps individuals manage negative thoughts and self-doubt by focusing on learning and development rather than perceived limitations.

- **Practice:** Use cognitive reframing techniques to challenge negative thoughts, focus on progress, and cultivate self-compassion.

5. Strategies for Cultivating a Growth Mindset

Set Growth-Oriented Goals:

- **Strategy:** Set goals that emphasize learning and improvement rather than solely focusing on outcomes. Establish goals that challenge you and encourage skill development.

- **Practice:** Define goals that involve acquiring new skills, overcoming challenges, and embracing opportunities for growth.

Embrace Challenges and Learn from Failure:

- **Strategy:** View challenges and failures as opportunities for growth and learning. Adopt a mindset that values effort and perseverance over immediate success.

- **Practice:** Approach setbacks with curiosity, analyze what can be learned, and apply insights to future endeavors.

Seek Feedback and Reflect:

- **Strategy:** Actively seek feedback from others and reflect on personal experiences to gain insights and improve. Use feedback as a tool for growth rather than criticism.

- **Practice:** Request feedback from mentors, peers, or colleagues, and reflect on how to incorporate suggestions into personal development.

Promote a Growth Mindset Environment:

- **Strategy:** Create an environment that encourages a growth mindset by fostering a culture of learning, experimentation, and support. Surround yourself with people who inspire and support your growth.

- **Practice:** Engage in activities and communities that promote learning and growth. Encourage and support others in their growth journey.

6. Integrating a Growth Mindset into Daily Life

Adopt a Positive Attitude:

- **Integration:** Maintain a positive attitude towards challenges and setbacks. Focus on learning and growth rather than dwelling on difficulties.

- **Practice:** Use affirmations, visualization, and positive self-talk to reinforce a growth mindset and foster optimism.

Celebrate Progress and Achievements:

- **Integration:** Recognize and celebrate progress and achievements, no matter how small. Acknowledge the effort and learning involved in reaching milestones.

- **Practice:** Track your progress, celebrate successes, and reflect on the growth and development achieved.

Cultivate Lifelong Learning:

- **Integration:** Continuously seek opportunities for learning and personal development. Embrace new experiences and challenges as part of a lifelong growth journey.

- **Practice:** Pursue educational courses, hobbies, and experiences that contribute to personal growth and development.

Cultivating a growth mindset is essential for lifelong wellness as it fosters resilience, adaptability, and continuous improvement. By embracing challenges, learning from experiences, and focusing on growth, individuals can enhance their physical, emotional, and mental well-being. Strategies such as setting growth-oriented goals, seeking feedback, and creating a supportive environment contribute to developing and maintaining a growth mindset. Integrating a growth mindset into daily life supports overall wellness and empowers individuals to navigate life's challenges with optimism and confidence.

Strategies for Overcoming Negative Thoughts and Emotions

Negative thoughts and emotions can significantly impact mental well-being and overall quality of life. However, with effective strategies, it is possible to manage and overcome these challenges, leading to improved emotional health and resilience. Here's a comprehensive guide to strategies for overcoming negative thoughts and emotions:

1. Identify and Challenge Negative Thoughts

Recognize Negative Thinking Patterns:

- **Technique:** Start by becoming aware of your negative thought patterns. Common types include all-or-nothing thinking, overgeneralization, and catastrophizing.

- **Practice:** Pay attention to your thoughts, especially during stressful situations. Notice recurring negative thoughts or automatic reactions.

Challenge Negative Thoughts:

- **Technique:** Question the validity of your negative thoughts. Ask yourself whether there is evidence supporting these thoughts or if they are based on assumptions or distortions.

- **Practice:** Use cognitive restructuring to reframe negative thoughts. For example, change "I always fail" to "I may face challenges, but I can learn and improve."

Replace with Positive or Neutral Thoughts:

- **Technique:** Substitute negative thoughts with more balanced, positive, or neutral ones. Focus on realistic and constructive alternatives.

- **Practice:** When you catch yourself thinking negatively, consciously replace those thoughts with positive affirmations or realistic observations. For example, instead of thinking "I can't do anything right," think "I have faced challenges before and overcome them."

2. Practice Mindfulness and Acceptance

Engage in Mindfulness Meditation:

- **Technique:** Mindfulness involves paying attention to the present moment without judgment. It helps in observing thoughts and emotions without becoming overwhelmed by them.

- **Practice:** Set aside time each day for mindfulness meditation. Focus on your breath and observe your thoughts and feelings as they arise, without reacting to them.

Practice Acceptance:

- **Technique:** Acceptance involves acknowledging and embracing negative thoughts and emotions rather than trying to suppress or deny them.

- **Practice:** Use acceptance techniques to observe negative thoughts and emotions without judgment. Remind yourself that it is okay to experience these feelings and that they are a natural part of life.

Use Grounding Techniques:

- **Technique:** Grounding techniques help bring your focus back to the present moment and away from negative thoughts or overwhelming emotions.

- **Practice:** Use grounding exercises such as deep breathing, progressive muscle relaxation, or focusing on physical sensations (e.g., feeling the texture of an object).

3. Engage in Self-Care and Stress Management

Prioritize Self-Care Activities:

- **Technique:** Self-care involves engaging in activities that promote well-being and relaxation. It helps in managing stress and improving mood.

- **Practice:** Incorporate self-care activities such as exercise, hobbies, spending time with loved ones, or engaging in creative pursuits into your routine.

Manage Stress Effectively:

- **Technique:** Stress management techniques help reduce the impact of stress on negative thinking and emotions. Common techniques include relaxation exercises, time management, and setting boundaries.

- **Practice:** Use stress reduction methods such as deep breathing exercises, yoga, or progressive muscle relaxation to manage stress levels.

Maintain a Healthy Lifestyle:

- **Technique:** A healthy lifestyle supports emotional well-being and resilience. This includes balanced nutrition, regular physical activity, and adequate sleep.

- **Practice:** Adopt healthy eating habits, engage in regular exercise, and ensure you get sufficient rest each night.

4. Seek Support and Build Resilience

Reach Out for Support:

- **Technique:** Talking to trusted friends, family members, or mental health professionals can provide support and perspective on negative thoughts and emotions.

- **Practice:** Share your feelings and experiences with someone you trust. Seek professional help if needed, such as counseling or therapy.

Build Emotional Resilience:

- **Technique:** Resilience involves developing the ability to bounce back from adversity and manage stress effectively. It is strengthened through positive coping strategies and support systems.

- **Practice:** Build resilience by setting realistic goals, developing problem-solving skills, and maintaining a supportive network of friends and family.

Engage in Positive Activities:

- **Technique:** Engaging in activities that bring joy and satisfaction can counteract negative emotions and foster a positive mindset.

- **Practice:** Participate in activities that you enjoy, such as hobbies, social events, or volunteer work. Focus on experiences that uplift and energize you.

5. Adopt Cognitive-Behavioral Techniques

Use Cognitive-Behavioral Strategies:

- **Technique:** Cognitive-behavioral therapy (CBT) techniques help in identifying and changing negative thought patterns and behaviors. They are effective in managing anxiety, depression, and stress.

- **Practice:** Apply CBT techniques such as thought records, behavioral experiments, and exposure exercises to address negative thoughts and emotions.

Implement Behavioral Activation:

- **Technique:** Behavioral activation involves engaging in activities that are meaningful and enjoyable to counteract negative emotions and improve mood.

- **Practice:** Schedule and participate in activities that align with your values and interests. Focus on activities that provide a sense of accomplishment and satisfaction.

Develop Problem-Solving Skills:

- **Technique:** Effective problem-solving skills help in addressing issues that contribute to negative thoughts and emotions. It involves identifying solutions and taking actionable steps.

- **Practice:** Use problem-solving techniques to address specific challenges or stressors. Break problems into manageable steps and develop strategies for resolution.

6. Foster a Growth Mindset

Embrace Challenges as Opportunities:

- **Technique:** Viewing challenges as opportunities for growth and learning can shift your perspective on negative experiences.

- **Practice:** Approach challenges with curiosity and a willingness to learn. Focus on the potential for personal growth and development.

Cultivate Self-Compassion:

- **Technique:** Self-compassion involves treating yourself with kindness and understanding, especially during difficult times.

- **Practice:** Practice self-compassion by speaking to yourself with kindness, acknowledging your struggles, and offering yourself support and encouragement.

Celebrate Small Wins:

- **Technique:** Recognizing and celebrating small achievements can boost confidence and counteract negative thoughts.

- **Practice:** Acknowledge and celebrate your progress, no matter how small. Reflect on your accomplishments and the effort involved.

Overcoming negative thoughts and emotions involves a multifaceted approach that includes identifying and challenging negative thinking patterns, practicing mindfulness and acceptance, engaging in self-care, seeking support, and adopting cognitive-behavioral techniques. By incorporating these strategies into daily life, individuals can manage and transform negative thoughts and emotions, leading to improved emotional well-being and resilience. Embracing a growth mindset, building emotional resilience, and fostering self-compassion are integral components of this journey towards a more positive and fulfilling life.

Chapter 9: E – Empower

Taking Control of Your Health Journey

Taking control of your health journey involves actively engaging in decisions and actions that impact your well-being. It requires self-awareness, proactive strategies, and a commitment to personal health goals. Here's a comprehensive guide to taking control of your health journey:

1. Set Clear and Achievable Health Goals

Define Your Objectives:

- **Technique:** Establish specific, measurable, attainable, relevant, and time-bound (SMART) goals related to your health. This provides clarity and direction for your health journey.

- **Practice:** Set goals such as "I will exercise for 30 minutes, five times a week" or "I will reduce my sugar intake by 50% over the next three months." Ensure that these goals align with your overall health priorities.

Create a Plan of Action:

- **Technique:** Develop a detailed plan outlining the steps needed to achieve your health goals. This includes identifying resources, setting milestones, and scheduling activities.

- **Practice:** Break down your goals into manageable steps. For example, if your goal is to improve your diet, start by planning weekly meals, grocery shopping for healthy foods, and learning new recipes.

Monitor and Adjust Goals:

- **Technique:** Regularly review your progress and adjust your goals and plan as needed. This ensures that your health journey remains dynamic and responsive to your evolving needs.

- **Practice:** Use tools such as journals, apps, or spreadsheets to track your progress. Reflect on what is working and what may need adjustment. Be flexible and make necessary changes to stay on track.

2. Adopt a Proactive Approach to Health

Educate Yourself:

- **Technique:** Gain knowledge about health topics relevant to your goals, such as nutrition, exercise, mental health, and disease prevention. Understanding the science behind health can inform your decisions and actions.

- **Practice:** Read books, attend workshops, or consult with healthcare professionals to enhance your understanding of health-related issues. Stay informed about new research and trends in health and wellness.

Engage in Preventive Health Measures:

- **Technique:** Take proactive steps to prevent health issues before they arise. This includes regular screenings, vaccinations, and maintaining a healthy lifestyle.

- **Practice:** Schedule and attend routine medical check-ups, screenings, and vaccinations. Incorporate preventive measures into your daily routine, such as using sunscreen, practicing good hygiene, and managing stress.

Incorporate Healthy Habits:

- **Technique:** Develop and maintain habits that support your overall health. This includes balanced nutrition, regular physical activity, adequate sleep, and stress management.

- **Practice:** Create a daily or weekly routine that includes healthy habits. For example, plan balanced meals, schedule workouts, establish a sleep routine, and incorporate relaxation techniques into your day.

3. Build a Support System

Seek Professional Guidance:

- **Technique:** Work with healthcare professionals, such as doctors, dietitians, and fitness trainers, to receive expert advice and support tailored to your individual needs.

- **Practice:** Schedule consultations with healthcare providers to discuss your health goals, get personalized recommendations, and address any concerns. Follow their advice and utilize their expertise to enhance your health journey.

Build a Support Network:

- **Technique:** Surround yourself with supportive individuals who encourage and motivate you on your health journey. This includes friends, family, and support groups.

- **Practice:** Share your health goals with trusted individuals who can offer encouragement and accountability. Join health-related communities or support groups to connect with others who share similar goals and experiences.

Engage in Social Support:

- **Technique:** Participate in social activities and relationships that promote well-being and provide emotional support. Positive social interactions can enhance motivation and overall health.

- **Practice:** Engage in activities with friends and family that promote a healthy lifestyle, such as group exercise classes, cooking healthy meals together, or participating in wellness challenges.

4. Empower Yourself with Knowledge and Resources

Utilize Health Resources:

- **Technique:** Access and use available resources to support your health journey. This includes educational materials, health apps, and community programs.

- **Practice:** Explore and use health apps that track your progress, offer fitness routines, or provide nutritional guidance. Take advantage of community resources such as wellness programs, fitness classes, or health fairs.

Stay Informed and Adapt:

- **Technique:** Continuously educate yourself and adapt your health plan based on new information and changes in your health status. Staying informed helps you make better decisions and stay proactive.

- **Practice:** Regularly review and update your knowledge about health trends and recommendations. Be open to adjusting your health plan based on new insights, research, or feedback from healthcare professionals.

Develop Self-Awareness:

- **Technique:** Cultivate self-awareness to understand your body's needs, preferences, and responses. This helps in making informed decisions and addressing any issues that arise.

- **Practice:** Pay attention to how your body reacts to different foods, exercises, and stressors. Reflect on your emotional and physical well-being to identify areas for improvement and make necessary adjustments.

5. Overcome Obstacles and Stay Motivated

Identify and Address Barriers:

- **Technique:** Recognize potential obstacles that may hinder your progress and develop strategies to overcome them. Common barriers include time constraints, lack of motivation, or conflicting priorities.

- **Practice:** Identify specific challenges you face and create actionable solutions. For example, if time is an issue, plan short, effective workouts or meal prep in advance to stay on track.

Maintain Motivation:

- **Technique:** Use motivational strategies to stay focused and committed to your health goals. This includes setting rewards, tracking progress, and celebrating achievements.

- **Practice:** Set small, achievable milestones and reward yourself for reaching them. Keep a progress journal or visual tracker to stay motivated and remind yourself of the positive changes you're making.

Adapt and Be Flexible:

- **Technique:** Be flexible and adaptable in your approach to health. Life circumstances and goals may change, and it's important to adjust your plan accordingly.

- **Practice:** Review and revise your health goals and plan as needed. Embrace flexibility by adapting to new situations or challenges and finding alternative solutions to maintain your progress.

Taking control of your health journey involves setting clear goals, adopting proactive health measures, building a support system, utilizing resources, and staying motivated. By actively engaging in decisions and actions that impact your well-being, you empower yourself to achieve and maintain optimal health. Embrace the process of continuous learning and self-improvement, and be adaptable in the face of challenges. Taking control of your health is a dynamic and ongoing journey, and with dedication and commitment, you can achieve lasting well-being and a fulfilling life.

Building Confidence in Your Ability to Heal

Building confidence in your ability to heal is crucial for overcoming health challenges and achieving lasting wellness. It involves developing a positive mindset, trusting in your body's natural capacity for recovery, and actively engaging in practices that support healing. Here's a comprehensive guide to building confidence in your ability to heal:

1. Recognize Your Body's Innate Healing Abilities

Understand the Body's Natural Healing Processes:

- **Technique:** Learn about how the body heals itself through processes such as inflammation, tissue repair, and immune response. This understanding reinforces your belief in your body's ability to recover.

- **Practice:** Read reputable sources about the body's natural healing mechanisms. Recognize that many common illnesses and injuries are self-limiting and improve over time with minimal intervention.

Acknowledge Past Healing Experiences:

- **Technique:** Reflect on previous instances where you have successfully healed from illnesses or injuries. This helps build confidence by reminding you of your body's resilience.

- **Practice:** Keep a journal or record of past health challenges and recoveries. Review these records to see how your body managed to heal and the steps you took that contributed to your recovery.

2. Set Realistic and Achievable Health Goals

Define Clear and Attainable Goals:

- **Technique:** Set health goals that are realistic and achievable based on your current condition and resources. This helps create a sense of purpose and direction in your healing journey.

- **Practice:** Use the SMART criteria (Specific, Measurable, Achievable, Relevant, Time-bound) to set your health goals. For example, if you're recovering from an injury, a goal could be "Increase range of motion in my shoulder by 20% over the next six weeks through physical therapy exercises."

Break Goals into Manageable Steps:

- **Technique:** Divide larger health goals into smaller, manageable tasks. This approach makes the process less overwhelming and provides a sense of accomplishment as you progress.

- **Practice:** Create a step-by-step plan for achieving your health goals. If your goal is to improve overall fitness, start with smaller steps like incorporating daily walks or gradually increasing exercise intensity.

3. Cultivate a Positive Mindset

Practice Positive Self-Talk:

- **Technique:** Replace negative or self-doubting thoughts with positive affirmations and encouraging self-talk. This helps reinforce your belief in your ability to heal.

- **Practice:** Use affirmations such as "I am strong and capable of healing" or "Every day, I am getting better." Repeat these affirmations regularly to foster a positive mindset.

Visualize Successful Healing:

- **Technique:** Use visualization techniques to imagine yourself successfully recovering and achieving your health goals. Visualization helps create a mental image of success and enhances motivation.

- **Practice:** Spend a few minutes each day visualizing yourself in a state of complete health and well-being. Imagine the steps you took and the positive outcomes of your healing process.

Focus on Progress, Not Perfection:

- **Technique:** Shift your focus from achieving perfection to recognizing and celebrating progress. Acknowledging small improvements boosts confidence and maintains motivation.

- **Practice:** Track your progress and celebrate milestones, no matter how small. For example, if you're working on improving your diet, celebrate each successful meal or healthy choice you make.

4. Engage in Supportive Practices

Adopt Healthy Lifestyle Habits:

- **Technique:** Engage in lifestyle habits that support healing, such as balanced nutrition, regular exercise, and adequate sleep. These practices contribute to overall well-being and enhance your body's ability to recover.

- **Practice:** Follow a balanced diet rich in nutrients, engage in regular physical activity suited to your condition, and ensure you get sufficient rest each night. Incorporate relaxation techniques to manage stress effectively.

Seek Professional Guidance:

- **Technique:** Work with healthcare professionals who can provide personalized advice and support for your healing journey. Their expertise helps build confidence in the effectiveness of your healing plan.

- **Practice:** Consult with doctors, nutritionists, or therapists as needed. Follow their recommendations and trust their guidance to support your recovery process.

Build a Support Network:

- **Technique:** Surround yourself with supportive individuals who encourage and motivate you. A positive support network reinforces your belief in your ability to heal.

- **Practice:** Share your health goals with friends and family. Seek support from those who uplift and encourage you. Consider joining support groups related to your health condition for additional encouragement.

5. Address and Overcome Self-Doubt

Identify and Challenge Self-Doubt:

- **Technique:** Recognize and address self-doubt or negative beliefs about your ability to heal. Challenge these thoughts by seeking evidence of your strengths and past successes.

- **Practice:** When self-doubt arises, ask yourself for evidence that contradicts these negative beliefs. Remind yourself of your past successes and the positive steps you are taking towards recovery.

Develop Resilience Through Problem-Solving:

- **Technique:** Strengthen your problem-solving skills to address challenges and setbacks effectively. Developing resilience helps you maintain confidence in your ability to overcome obstacles.

- **Practice:** Use problem-solving techniques to address any difficulties you encounter. Break down problems into smaller parts, generate potential solutions, and implement strategies to overcome challenges.

Accept and Learn from Setbacks:

- **Technique:** Accept that setbacks may occur and view them as opportunities for learning and growth. Resilience involves bouncing back from setbacks and continuing to move forward.

- **Practice:** When faced with setbacks, reflect on what you can learn from the experience. Adjust your plan as needed and focus on the steps you can take to continue progressing towards your goals.

6. Create a Sustainable Healing Plan

Develop a Comprehensive Healing Plan:

- **Technique:** Create a holistic and sustainable plan that addresses various aspects of health, including physical, emotional, and mental well-being. A well-rounded plan enhances overall recovery.

- **Practice:** Include elements such as nutrition, exercise, stress management, and self-care in your healing plan. Regularly review and adjust your plan based on your progress and evolving needs.

Stay Committed and Consistent:

- **Technique:** Consistency is key to achieving long-term healing and maintaining confidence. Stay committed to your plan and make adjustments as needed to stay on track.

- **Practice:** Establish a routine for implementing your healing plan. Set reminders or create a schedule to help you stay consistent with your practices and goals.

Reflect and Adapt:

- **Technique:** Regularly reflect on your progress and adapt your plan based on your experiences and feedback. Continuous reflection helps you stay aligned with your goals and adjust to changing circumstances.

- **Practice:** Schedule regular check-ins with yourself to assess your progress. Make any necessary adjustments to your plan and celebrate your successes along the way.

Building confidence in your ability to heal involves recognizing your body's natural healing capabilities, setting achievable goals, cultivating a positive mindset, engaging in supportive practices, addressing self-doubt, and creating a sustainable healing plan. By actively participating in your health journey and focusing on progress, you empower yourself to overcome challenges and achieve lasting well-being. Embrace the process with patience and persistence, and trust in your body's ability to recover and thrive.

Creating a Sustainable Wellness Plan

Creating a sustainable wellness plan is crucial for maintaining long-term health and well-being. This plan should be practical, adaptable, and tailored to your individual needs, helping you integrate healthy practices into your daily life. Here's a comprehensive guide to developing a wellness plan that promotes lasting health:

1. Assess Your Current Health and Wellness

Conduct a Personal Health Assessment:

- **Technique:** Evaluate your current physical, mental, and emotional health to identify areas that need improvement and set clear goals for your wellness plan.

- **Practice:** Use health assessments such as self-surveys or questionnaires to evaluate factors like nutrition, physical fitness, stress levels, and sleep quality. Consider consulting a healthcare professional for a more comprehensive assessment.

Identify Your Health Goals:

- **Technique:** Define specific, measurable, achievable, relevant, and time-bound (SMART) goals based on your assessment. This helps create a clear direction for your wellness plan.

- **Practice:** Set goals such as "Improve cardiovascular health by incorporating 30 minutes of exercise five times a week" or "Enhance sleep quality by establishing a consistent bedtime routine."

2. Design a Comprehensive Wellness Plan

Incorporate Key Wellness Components:

- **Technique:** Include essential elements such as nutrition, physical activity, stress management, and sleep in your wellness plan. A holistic approach ensures that all aspects of health are addressed.

- **Practice:** Develop a plan that includes balanced meal plans, regular exercise routines, stress reduction techniques, and healthy sleep habits. Ensure each component is realistic and aligns with your goals.

Create a Daily Routine:

- **Technique:** Establish a daily routine that incorporates wellness practices into your life. Consistency helps reinforce healthy habits and makes them a natural part of your day.

- **Practice:** Design a schedule that includes time for meal preparation, exercise, relaxation, and sleep. Use tools like planners or digital apps to organize and track your daily activities.

3. Set Up Tracking and Evaluation Systems

Monitor Your Progress:

- **Technique:** Regularly track your progress to assess the effectiveness of your wellness plan and make adjustments as needed. This helps ensure that you stay on track and achieve your goals.

- **Practice:** Use journals, apps, or charts to monitor key indicators such as exercise frequency, dietary intake, stress levels, and sleep patterns. Review your progress weekly or monthly.

Evaluate and Adjust Your Plan:

- **Technique:** Periodically evaluate the outcomes of your wellness plan and adjust strategies based on your experiences and results. Flexibility allows you to address challenges and optimize your plan.

- **Practice:** Set aside time for regular evaluations, such as monthly reviews, to assess your progress and make any necessary changes. Adjust your goals or strategies based on what is working well and what needs improvement.

4. Incorporate Healthy Eating Practices

Develop a Balanced Nutrition Plan:

- **Technique:** Create a meal plan that includes a variety of nutrient-dense foods to support overall health. Focus on whole foods and minimize processed food consumption.

- **Practice:** Plan meals and snacks that incorporate vegetables, fruits, whole grains, lean proteins, and healthy fats. Use meal planning tools or apps to organize your weekly food intake.

Ensure Adequate Hydration:

- **Technique:** Maintain proper hydration by drinking sufficient water throughout the day. Hydration is essential for overall health and supports bodily functions.

- **Practice:** Set reminders to drink water regularly and keep a water bottle with you. Aim for about 8 cups (2 liters) of water daily, adjusting based on activity level and individual needs.

5. Integrate Physical Activity

Choose Enjoyable Forms of Exercise:

- **Technique:** Select physical activities that you enjoy to increase the likelihood of sticking with your exercise routine. Enjoyable activities make exercise more sustainable.

- **Practice:** Explore various forms of exercise such as walking, jogging, swimming, cycling, or yoga. Choose activities that you find enjoyable and that fit your fitness level.

Create a Structured Exercise Routine:

- **Technique:** Develop a structured exercise routine that includes a mix of cardiovascular, strength, flexibility, and balance exercises. Aim for at least 150 minutes of moderate-intensity exercise per week.

- **Practice:** Schedule exercise sessions into your weekly routine, incorporating different types of workouts. Use fitness apps or hire a personal trainer to help design and stick to your routine.

6. Implement Stress Management Techniques

Adopt Relaxation Practices:

- **Technique:** Integrate relaxation techniques such as deep breathing, progressive muscle relaxation, or guided imagery to manage stress effectively.

- **Practice:** Dedicate time each day to practice relaxation techniques. Use guided meditation apps or attend relaxation classes to enhance your stress management skills.

Establish Healthy Boundaries:

- **Technique:** Set boundaries to manage stress and avoid burnout. This includes balancing work and personal life, learning to say no, and prioritizing self-care.

- **Practice:** Create boundaries around work hours, personal time, and social commitments. Practice assertiveness in managing your time and responsibilities to reduce stress.

7. Enhance Sleep Quality

Develop a Consistent Sleep Schedule:

- **Technique:** Establish a consistent sleep schedule by going to bed and waking up at the same time each day. Consistency supports healthy sleep patterns.

- **Practice:** Set a bedtime routine that helps signal to your body that it's time to wind down. Avoid screens and stimulating activities before bed to improve sleep quality.

Create a Restful Sleep Environment:

- **Technique:** Optimize your sleep environment to promote restful sleep. This includes a comfortable mattress, a dark, quiet room, and a cool temperature.

- **Practice:** Make adjustments to your bedroom environment to enhance sleep, such as using blackout curtains, white noise machines, or cooling fans.

8. Foster Emotional and Mental Well-Being

Cultivate Positive Relationships:

- **Technique:** Build and maintain positive relationships with family, friends, and support networks. Social connections play a vital role in emotional well-being.

- **Practice:** Engage in activities that strengthen your relationships, such as spending quality time with loved ones, participating in community events, and seeking support when needed.

Practice Self-Compassion:

- **Technique:** Treat yourself with kindness and understanding, especially during challenging times. Self-compassion helps build resilience and reduces stress.

- **Practice:** Use positive self-talk and self-care practices to nurture yourself. Recognize your efforts and achievements, and be gentle with yourself during setbacks.

9. Embrace Lifelong Learning and Growth

Stay Informed About Health and Wellness:

- **Technique:** Continuously educate yourself about health and wellness topics to stay informed and make better choices for your well-being.

- **Practice:** Read books, attend workshops, and follow reputable sources on health and wellness. Stay curious and open to new information and practices.

Adapt and Evolve Your Plan:

- **Technique:** Be flexible and willing to adapt your wellness plan as your needs and circumstances change. An evolving plan ensures continued relevance and effectiveness.

- **Practice:** Regularly review and update your wellness plan based on changes in your health status, goals, and lifestyle. Embrace new practices and adjust strategies as needed.

Creating a sustainable wellness plan involves assessing your current health, designing a comprehensive and adaptable plan, tracking progress, and integrating key wellness components. By incorporating healthy eating, physical activity, stress management, and other essential practices, you can develop a holistic approach to well-being that supports long-term health. Stay committed, flexible, and proactive in your wellness journey, and enjoy the benefits of a healthier and more balanced life.

PART TWO: PRACTICAL APPLICATIONS

Chapter 10: Integrating the SUSTAIN ME Principles

Creating a Personalized Wellness Plan

A personalized wellness plan is a tailored approach to achieving optimal health and well-being, taking into account your unique needs, goals, and lifestyle. It provides a structured framework for integrating healthy practices into your daily routine, helping you to stay motivated and make sustainable changes. Here's how to create a personalized wellness plan that is both effective and adaptable:

1. Assess Your Current Health Status

Conduct a Comprehensive Health Assessment:

- **Technique:** Begin by evaluating your current physical, mental, and emotional health. Identify any existing health conditions, lifestyle habits, and areas for improvement.

- **Practice:** Use self-assessment tools such as health questionnaires, fitness trackers, and dietary logs. Consider consulting a healthcare provider for a thorough health evaluation, including blood tests or other diagnostic measures.

Identify Your Wellness Goals:

- **Technique:** Define specific, achievable goals that align with your health needs and personal aspirations. Setting clear goals helps to focus your efforts and measure progress.

- **Practice:** Set SMART goals (Specific, Measurable, Achievable, Relevant, Time-bound) such as "Lose 10 pounds in 3 months" or "Improve flexibility by attending yoga classes twice a week." Ensure your goals are realistic and tailored to your current health status.

2. Design a Balanced Wellness Plan

Incorporate Key Components:

- **Technique:** Create a plan that includes various aspects of wellness such as nutrition, physical activity, stress management, sleep, and mental health. A well-rounded approach ensures that all areas of health are addressed.

- **Practice:** Develop a plan that incorporates balanced meal planning, regular exercise, relaxation techniques, and strategies for improving sleep and mental health. Tailor each component to fit your personal preferences and needs.

Create a Daily and Weekly Schedule:

- **Technique:** Organize your wellness plan into a structured daily and weekly routine. Consistent practices make it easier to integrate healthy habits into your life.

- **Practice:** Design a schedule that includes time for meal preparation, exercise, stress management activities, and sleep. Use tools like planners or digital apps to track and manage your routine effectively.

3. Develop a Nutrition Plan

Design a Balanced Diet:

- **Technique:** Create a meal plan that includes a variety of nutrient-dense foods to meet your dietary needs. Focus on whole foods and balanced macronutrients.

- **Practice:** Plan meals that include vegetables, fruits, lean proteins, whole grains, and healthy fats. Avoid excessive processed foods and sugary snacks. Use meal planning apps or consult a nutritionist for guidance.

Incorporate Hydration:

- **Technique:** Ensure adequate hydration by drinking enough water throughout the day. Proper hydration supports overall health and bodily functions.

- **Practice:** Aim to drink at least 8 cups (2 liters) of water daily. Adjust your intake based on activity level, climate, and individual needs. Use reminders or apps to help you stay on track.

4. Integrate Physical Activity

Choose Activities You Enjoy:

- **Technique:** Select forms of exercise that you find enjoyable and motivating. Engaging in activities you like increases the likelihood of sticking with your routine.

- **Practice:** Explore different types of exercise such as walking, cycling, swimming, or dance. Find activities that align with your interests and fitness level.

Create an Exercise Routine:

- **Technique:** Develop a structured exercise plan that includes a mix of cardiovascular, strength, flexibility, and balance exercises. Aim for a balanced approach to fitness.

- **Practice:** Schedule regular workouts into your week, such as 150 minutes of moderate-intensity exercise or 75 minutes of vigorous exercise per week. Incorporate strength training exercises at least twice a week.

5. Implement Stress Management Strategies

Incorporate Relaxation Techniques:

- **Technique:** Include stress management practices such as deep breathing, meditation, or progressive muscle relaxation. These techniques help reduce stress and promote mental clarity.

- **Practice:** Dedicate time each day to practice relaxation techniques. Use guided meditation apps or attend stress management workshops to enhance your skills.

Set Boundaries and Prioritize Self-Care:

- **Technique:** Establish boundaries to manage stress and prevent burnout. Prioritize self-care and balance work, personal life, and relaxation.

- **Practice:** Create boundaries around work hours and personal time. Engage in activities that promote relaxation and self-care, such as hobbies, reading, or spending time with loved ones.

6. Enhance Sleep Quality

Develop a Consistent Sleep Routine:

- **Technique:** Establish a regular sleep schedule by going to bed and waking up at the same time each day. Consistency supports healthy sleep patterns.

- **Practice:** Set a bedtime routine that promotes relaxation, such as reading or taking a warm bath. Avoid screens and stimulating activities before bed.

Optimize Your Sleep Environment:

- **Technique:** Create a restful sleep environment by making adjustments to your bedroom. A conducive sleep environment improves sleep quality.

- **Practice:** Ensure your bedroom is dark, quiet, and cool. Invest in a comfortable mattress and pillows, and consider using blackout curtains or white noise machines.

7. Address Mental and Emotional Well-Being

Foster Positive Relationships:

- **Technique:** Build and maintain positive relationships with family, friends, and support networks. Social connections contribute to emotional well-being.

- **Practice:** Engage in activities that strengthen relationships, such as spending quality time with loved ones and participating in social events.

Practice Self-Compassion:

- **Technique:** Treat yourself with kindness and understanding, especially during challenging times. Self-compassion helps build resilience and reduces stress.

- **Practice:** Use positive self-talk and self-care practices. Acknowledge your efforts and achievements, and be gentle with yourself during setbacks.

8. Monitor and Adjust Your Plan

Track Your Progress:

- **Technique:** Regularly monitor your progress to evaluate the effectiveness of your wellness plan and make adjustments as needed.

- **Practice:** Use journals, apps, or charts to track key indicators such as exercise frequency, dietary intake, stress levels, and sleep quality. Review your progress regularly.

Evaluate and Adapt Your Plan:

- **Technique:** Periodically assess the outcomes of your wellness plan and adjust strategies based on your experiences and results.

- **Practice:** Set aside time for regular evaluations, such as monthly reviews, to assess your progress and make necessary changes. Adjust your goals or strategies based on what is working well and what needs improvement.

9. Seek Professional Guidance

Consult Healthcare Professionals:

- **Technique:** Seek guidance from healthcare providers, nutritionists, or fitness experts for personalized recommendations and support.

- **Practice:** Schedule regular check-ups with your healthcare provider to monitor your health and receive professional advice. Consult a nutritionist or personal trainer for tailored recommendations.

Stay Informed About Wellness Trends:

- **Technique:** Keep up-to-date with the latest research and trends in health and wellness to enhance your plan and make informed decisions.

- **Practice:** Read books, attend workshops, and follow reputable sources on health and wellness. Stay open to new information and practices that may benefit your well-being.

Creating a personalized wellness plan involves assessing your current health, setting achievable goals, and integrating various aspects of wellness into your daily routine. By incorporating nutrition, physical activity, stress management, sleep, and mental health practices, you can develop a comprehensive plan that supports your overall well-being. Regular monitoring and adjustments ensure that your plan remains effective and relevant to your needs. Embrace the journey towards better health with commitment and flexibility, and enjoy the benefits of a healthier, more balanced life.

Tracking Progress and Making Adjustments

Tracking progress and making adjustments is a crucial aspect of maintaining a personalized wellness plan. It ensures that you stay on course towards your health goals and allows for the optimization of strategies based on real-time feedback. Here's how to effectively monitor your progress and make necessary adjustments to enhance your wellness journey:

1. Establish Key Metrics and Indicators

Identify Relevant Metrics:

- **Technique:** Determine the key metrics that will help you measure progress towards your wellness goals. These metrics should align with the specific areas of your plan, such as physical fitness, dietary habits, mental health, and overall well-being.

- **Practice:** Metrics may include weight, body measurements, fitness levels, sleep quality, stress levels, mood, and dietary intake. Choose metrics that provide meaningful insights into your progress and health status.

Set Baseline Measurements:

- **Technique:** Record initial measurements to establish a baseline. This allows you to track changes and evaluate progress over time.

- **Practice:** Document your starting values for each metric, such as your current weight, daily steps, sleep duration, and dietary patterns. Use this baseline as a reference point for future comparisons.

2. Regular Monitoring and Evaluation

Track Your Progress Consistently:

- **Technique:** Implement a system for regular monitoring of your wellness metrics. Consistent tracking provides a clear picture of your progress and helps identify trends or areas needing adjustment.

- **Practice:** Use tools such as health and fitness apps, journals, or spreadsheets to log your data. Set a routine for checking and recording your metrics, such as weekly or monthly.

Review and Analyze Data:

- **Technique:** Regularly review and analyze the data you've collected to assess progress towards your goals. Look for patterns, improvements, or areas where you may be falling short.

- **Practice:** Analyze trends in your metrics, such as changes in weight, fitness levels, or stress levels. Identify any correlations between your efforts and outcomes to determine what is working well and what needs improvement.

3. Make Informed Adjustments

Adjust Based on Feedback:

- **Technique:** Use the insights gained from tracking to make informed adjustments to your wellness plan. This ensures that your plan remains effective and relevant to your needs.

- **Practice:** If you notice that you're not meeting your goals or experiencing challenges, consider modifying your approach. For example, if weight loss is slower than expected, review and adjust your diet and exercise routines.

Set New Goals and Targets:

- **Technique:** As you progress, set new goals or targets to continue challenging yourself and maintaining motivation. Adjusting your goals helps to ensure ongoing progress and prevent stagnation.

- **Practice:** Based on your progress, set short-term and long-term goals that build on your achievements. For instance, if you've successfully incorporated regular exercise, set a new target for increasing your workout intensity or duration.

4. Address Challenges and Barriers

Identify Obstacles:

- **Technique:** Recognize any obstacles or barriers that may be hindering your progress. Addressing these challenges is essential for maintaining momentum and achieving your goals.

- **Practice:** Reflect on any difficulties you encounter, such as time constraints, lack of motivation, or dietary challenges. Identify specific issues that are affecting your progress and consider solutions or strategies to overcome them.

Develop Solutions and Strategies:

- **Technique:** Create actionable solutions and strategies to address the obstacles you've identified. This may involve modifying your plan, seeking support, or implementing new techniques.

- **Practice:** If time constraints are affecting your ability to exercise, explore ways to integrate shorter, more efficient workouts into your schedule. Consider seeking support from a coach, therapist, or support group if motivation is a challenge.

5. Seek Feedback and Support

Consult with Professionals:

- **Technique:** Seek feedback and guidance from healthcare professionals, nutritionists, or fitness experts to gain insights and recommendations for improvement.

- **Practice:** Schedule regular check-ins with professionals to review your progress and receive expert advice. Use their feedback to refine your wellness plan and address any concerns.

Engage with Support Networks:

- **Technique:** Connect with support networks, such as friends, family, or wellness communities, to share your progress and gain encouragement.

- **Practice:** Participate in support groups or online forums where you can discuss your experiences, share successes, and seek advice from others on similar wellness journeys.

6. Celebrate Successes and Reflect on Achievements

Acknowledge Milestones:

- **Technique:** Celebrate your successes and milestones along the way. Recognizing your achievements boosts motivation and reinforces positive behavior.

- **Practice:** Set small rewards for reaching specific goals, such as treating yourself to a new workout outfit or enjoying a relaxing day off. Reflect on your progress and the positive changes you've made.

Reflect on Your Journey:

- **Technique:** Periodically reflect on your wellness journey to evaluate what you've learned and how far you've come. This reflection helps to reinforce your commitment and identify areas for continued growth.

- **Practice:** Take time to journal or meditate on your experiences, achievements, and lessons learned. Use this reflection to inspire and motivate yourself as you continue your wellness journey.

Tracking progress and making adjustments is an ongoing process that requires attention, reflection, and flexibility. By establishing key metrics, monitoring progress, making informed adjustments, and addressing challenges, you can effectively manage your personalized wellness plan. Celebrate your successes, seek support when needed, and continuously refine your approach to ensure that you stay on track and achieve your health goals. Embrace the journey with commitment and openness, and enjoy the benefits of a well-balanced and evolving wellness plan.

Overcoming Common Challenges

Embarking on a wellness journey can present various challenges, but addressing these obstacles effectively can lead to long-term success and improved health. Understanding common challenges and implementing strategies to overcome them is crucial for maintaining motivation and achieving your goals. Here's how to tackle some of the most frequently encountered challenges:

1. Time Constraints

Challenge:

- Finding time to exercise, prepare healthy meals, and manage other wellness activities can be difficult amidst a busy schedule.

Strategies:

- **Prioritize and Schedule:** Allocate specific times for wellness activities in your daily or weekly schedule. Treat these appointments with the same importance as work meetings or social engagements.

- **Efficient Workouts:** Opt for shorter, high-intensity workouts if you have limited time. Even brief sessions can be effective when performed consistently.

- **Meal Prep:** Plan and prepare meals in advance to save time during the week. Batch cooking or using meal delivery services can streamline your food preparation process.

2. Lack of Motivation

Challenge:

- Maintaining motivation over the long term can be challenging, especially when progress slows or obstacles arise.

Strategies:

- **Set Clear Goals:** Establish specific, achievable goals and regularly review them to stay focused. Break larger goals into smaller milestones to maintain motivation and track progress.

- **Find Support:** Engage with a support network, such as friends, family, or a wellness community, to stay accountable and motivated. Sharing your journey with others can provide encouragement and inspiration.

- **Celebrate Successes:** Acknowledge and reward yourself for reaching milestones, no matter how small. Celebrating achievements can boost motivation and reinforce positive behavior.

3. Plateaus and Slow Progress

Challenge:

- Experiencing a plateau or slow progress can be frustrating and may lead to discouragement.

Strategies:

- **Reevaluate Your Plan:** Assess your current wellness plan and make adjustments if necessary. Changing your exercise routine, modifying your diet, or exploring new wellness practices can help break through plateaus.

- **Track Progress:** Keep detailed records of your progress and review them to identify patterns or areas needing improvement. Adjusting your approach based on this feedback can facilitate continued progress.

- **Seek Professional Guidance:** Consult with a healthcare provider, nutritionist, or fitness expert for personalized recommendations and strategies to overcome plateaus.

4. Difficulty with Habit Formation

Challenge:

- Establishing and maintaining new habits can be challenging, especially if you have a history of inconsistent behavior.

Strategies:

- **Start Small:** Begin with small, manageable changes that are easier to incorporate into your routine. Gradually build on these changes to establish more significant habits.

- **Use Triggers:** Create cues or triggers that remind you to engage in your new habits. For example, leave your workout clothes out as a visual reminder to exercise.

- **Build Routine:** Incorporate new habits into your daily routine to make them more automatic. Consistency is key to forming lasting habits.

5. Dealing with Setbacks

Challenge:

- Setbacks, such as illness, injury, or life events, can disrupt your wellness plan and affect your progress.

Strategies:

- **Adjust and Adapt:** Be flexible and adjust your plan as needed to accommodate setbacks. Modify your activities or goals to align with your current situation.

- **Practice Self-Compassion:** Approach setbacks with self-compassion and avoid self-criticism. Recognize that setbacks are a natural part of the journey and focus on moving forward.

- **Seek Support:** Reach out for support from friends, family, or professionals to help you navigate setbacks and stay on track.

6. Financial Constraints

Challenge:

- Limited financial resources can affect your ability to access certain wellness activities, such as gym memberships or specialty foods.

Strategies:

- **Utilize Free Resources:** Take advantage of free or low-cost wellness resources, such as online workout videos, community fitness classes, or public parks for exercise.

- **Budget for Wellness:** Prioritize wellness in your budget by allocating funds for essential items and activities. Look for discounts, deals, or affordable alternatives that fit your financial situation.

- **DIY Solutions:** Create your own wellness solutions, such as homemade meal plans or at-home workouts, to reduce costs while maintaining your wellness routine.

7. Balancing Wellness with Other Responsibilities

Challenge:

- Balancing wellness activities with work, family, and other responsibilities can be challenging and may lead to conflicts.

Strategies:

- **Integrate Wellness:** Find ways to integrate wellness activities into your daily life. For example, involve family members in physical activities or incorporate mindfulness practices into your workday.

- **Set Boundaries:** Establish clear boundaries to ensure that you have dedicated time for wellness without compromising other responsibilities. Communicate your needs with family or colleagues to gain their support.

- **Practice Flexibility:** Be flexible and adaptable with your wellness plan. Adjust your activities and goals to fit your schedule and priorities.

8. Overcoming Negative Self-Talk

Challenge:

- Negative self-talk and self-doubt can undermine your confidence and hinder your progress.

Strategies:

- **Challenge Negative Thoughts:** Identify and challenge negative thoughts by reframing them into positive and constructive statements. Focus on your strengths and achievements rather than perceived shortcomings.

- **Practice Positive Affirmations:** Use positive affirmations to reinforce your self-worth and build confidence. Regularly remind yourself of your capabilities and progress.

- **Seek Professional Help:** If negative self-talk persists and impacts your well-being, consider seeking support from a therapist or counselor to address underlying issues and build resilience.

Overcoming common challenges requires proactive strategies, flexibility, and persistence. By addressing obstacles such as time constraints, lack of motivation, plateaus, and financial constraints, you can maintain momentum and stay on track with your wellness plan. Embrace setbacks as opportunities for growth, seek support when needed, and practice self-compassion. With determination and a positive mindset, you can successfully navigate challenges and achieve your wellness goals.

Chapter 11: Herbal Remedies and Natural Solutions

An Introduction to Herbal Medicine

Herbal medicine, also known as botanical medicine or phytotherapy, is a practice that dates back thousands of years. It involves using plants or plant extracts to prevent and treat various ailments and to promote overall health. This natural approach to healing is grounded in the belief that plants have therapeutic properties that can address the root causes of health issues rather than merely alleviating symptoms. As modern medicine increasingly recognizes the value of holistic and integrative health practices, herbal medicine continues to gain popularity for its effectiveness, accessibility, and minimal side effects.

1. The History and Evolution of Herbal Medicine

Herbal medicine has been an integral part of human healthcare for millennia. Ancient civilizations, including those in Egypt, China, India, and Greece, used herbs to treat a wide range of conditions. For example, the ancient Egyptians used garlic for its antibacterial properties, while Traditional Chinese Medicine (TCM) has long relied on herbs like ginseng and ginger for their healing properties.

Over the centuries, knowledge of herbal medicine was passed down through generations, often within families or through apprenticeships with herbalists and traditional healers. In the Western world, herbal medicine was practiced by folk healers and midwives, and many modern pharmaceuticals are derived from these traditional remedies. For instance, aspirin was originally derived from willow bark, which was used for centuries to relieve pain and inflammation.

2. The Principles of Herbal Medicine

Herbal medicine is based on the principle that the body has an inherent ability to heal itself when supported by natural remedies. Unlike conventional medicine, which often focuses on treating symptoms, herbal medicine aims to address the underlying causes of illness by restoring balance to the body's systems. This holistic approach considers not just the physical symptoms but also the emotional, mental, and spiritual aspects of health.

Herbal medicine practitioners believe in the synergy of plant compounds, where the whole plant is often more effective than isolated active ingredients. This contrasts with pharmaceutical drugs, which typically focus on single active components. The use of whole plants or plant extracts allows for a more balanced and gentle treatment, minimizing the risk of side effects.

3. Common Forms of Herbal Medicine

Herbal medicine can be administered in various forms, depending on the condition being treated and the preferences of the patient. Some of the most common forms include:

- **Teas and Infusions:** Prepared by steeping herbs in hot water, teas and infusions are simple and effective ways to extract the medicinal properties of plants. They are commonly used for digestive issues, colds, and stress relief.

- **Tinctures:** These are concentrated liquid extracts made by soaking herbs in alcohol or vinegar. Tinctures are potent and convenient, allowing for easy dosage adjustments.

- **Capsules and Tablets:** These are convenient forms for those who prefer not to taste the herbs. Capsules contain powdered herbs, while tablets may contain extracts or whole herbs compressed into pill form.

- **Salves and Ointments:** Used topically, these are prepared by infusing herbs in oils or fats, which are then combined with beeswax or other thickening agents. They are commonly used for skin conditions, wounds, and muscle aches.

- **Essential Oils:** These are highly concentrated extracts obtained through distillation. Essential oils are typically used in aromatherapy or diluted for topical application.

- **Poultices and Compresses:** These involve applying whole herbs or their extracts directly to the skin to treat injuries, inflammation, or skin conditions.

4. The Role of Herbal Medicine in Modern Healthcare

In today's world, there is a growing interest in integrating herbal medicine with conventional medical practices. Many people are turning to herbal remedies to complement or replace pharmaceutical drugs, particularly for chronic conditions where conventional treatments may have limited efficacy or undesirable side effects. Herbal medicine offers a natural, sustainable approach to health that aligns with the body's healing processes.

Research into the efficacy of herbal medicine is expanding, with numerous studies supporting the use of specific herbs for conditions such as anxiety, insomnia, digestive disorders, and immune support. For example, St. John's Wort is widely studied for its antidepressant properties, while echinacea is recognized for its immune-boosting effects.

5. Safety and Considerations

While herbal medicine is generally safe, it is essential to approach it with caution and respect. Some herbs can interact with pharmaceutical drugs or may not be suitable for everyone, particularly pregnant women, children, or individuals with certain health conditions. It's important to consult with a qualified herbalist or healthcare provider before starting any herbal regimen.

Dosage and preparation methods are also crucial factors in the safety and effectiveness of herbal medicine. Overconsumption or improper use of certain herbs can lead to adverse effects. Additionally, the quality of herbs is vital, as contaminants or poor harvesting and processing practices can reduce their efficacy.

6. Getting Started with Herbal Medicine

For those new to herbal medicine, it's advisable to start with a few well-known and widely studied herbs. Some beginner-friendly herbs include:

- **Chamomile:** Known for its calming effects, chamomile is often used to relieve anxiety and improve sleep.

- **Peppermint:** This herb is commonly used for digestive issues and to relieve headaches.

- **Ginger:** Renowned for its anti-inflammatory and digestive properties, ginger is effective for nausea, motion sickness, and joint pain.

- **Lavender:** Often used in aromatherapy, lavender can help with relaxation, stress relief, and insomnia.

- **Echinacea:** This immune-boosting herb is commonly used to prevent or reduce the severity of colds and flu.

Herbal medicine offers a time-tested, natural approach to health and wellness that complements modern healthcare practices. By understanding the principles, forms, and safety considerations of herbal medicine, individuals can effectively incorporate these natural remedies into their health routines. Whether used for prevention, treatment, or overall well-being, herbal medicine provides a holistic path to nurturing and sustaining health.

Key Herbs for Common Ailments

Herbs have been used for centuries to treat a variety of common ailments, offering natural and often gentler alternatives to pharmaceutical drugs. While modern medicine has brought many advancements, the interest in herbal remedies continues to grow due to their effectiveness, minimal side effects, and holistic approach to healing. Understanding which herbs to use for specific conditions can empower individuals to manage their health naturally and effectively.

1. Herbs for Digestive Issues

Digestive problems, such as indigestion, bloating, and constipation, are common and can be effectively managed with herbal remedies.

- **Peppermint (Mentha piperita):** Peppermint is widely recognized for its ability to soothe the digestive system. Its antispasmodic properties help relax the muscles of the gastrointestinal tract, making it effective for relieving symptoms of irritable bowel syndrome (IBS) and indigestion. Peppermint tea is a simple way to enjoy its benefits.

- **Ginger (Zingiber officinale):** Ginger is a powerful anti-inflammatory and digestive aid. It can alleviate nausea, vomiting, and motion sickness, and is also used to treat bloating and indigestion. Fresh ginger can be added to meals, or ginger tea can be consumed to soothe the stomach.

- **Chamomile (Matricaria chamomilla):** Chamomile is known for its calming effects and is often used to ease digestive discomfort. It helps reduce gas, bloating, and stomach cramps, making it ideal for those with sensitive stomachs. Chamomile tea is a popular and gentle option for digestive relief.

- **Fennel (Foeniculum vulgare):** Fennel seeds are traditionally used to relieve bloating, gas, and indigestion. They have carminative properties that help expel gas from the digestive tract. Fennel tea or chewing fennel seeds after meals can aid digestion.

2. Herbs for Respiratory Health

Respiratory issues, such as colds, coughs, and asthma, can be managed with herbs that support lung function and boost the immune system.

- **Echinacea (Echinacea purpurea):** Echinacea is renowned for its immune-boosting properties. It is often used to prevent and treat the common cold and upper respiratory infections. Echinacea can be taken as a tea, tincture, or capsule.

- **Licorice Root (Glycyrrhiza glabra):** Licorice root has expectorant and soothing properties, making it useful for relieving coughs, sore throats, and bronchitis. It helps thin mucus and ease breathing. However, it should be used cautiously, especially in those with high blood pressure, as it can cause water retention.

- **Thyme (Thymus vulgaris):** Thyme has antimicrobial and expectorant properties, making it effective for treating coughs and respiratory infections. Thyme tea or a steam inhalation can help clear mucus and soothe the respiratory tract.

- **Mullein (Verbascum thapsus):** Mullein is known for its ability to support respiratory health. It helps soothe the lungs, reduce inflammation, and expel mucus. Mullein tea or tincture can be used for coughs, bronchitis, and asthma.

3. Herbs for Stress and Anxiety

Managing stress and anxiety is crucial for overall well-being, and certain herbs can help calm the mind and body naturally.

- **Ashwagandha (Withania somnifera):** Ashwagandha is an adaptogenic herb that helps the body cope with stress by balancing cortisol levels and supporting adrenal health. It is also known to reduce anxiety and improve mood. Ashwagandha can be taken as a powder, capsule, or tincture.

- **Valerian (Valeriana officinalis):** Valerian is a well-known herb for promoting relaxation and improving sleep. It is often used to reduce anxiety and tension. Valerian root can be consumed as a tea or in capsule form.

- **Lavender (Lavandula angustifolia):** Lavender is famous for its calming effects and is often used to alleviate anxiety, stress, and insomnia. Lavender essential oil can be used in aromatherapy, or lavender tea can be consumed for a soothing effect.

- **Lemon Balm (Melissa officinalis):** Lemon balm is a gentle herb that helps reduce stress and anxiety. It has a mild sedative effect, making it useful for promoting relaxation and improving sleep. Lemon balm tea is a popular way to enjoy its benefits.

4. Herbs for Pain and Inflammation

Chronic pain and inflammation can significantly impact quality of life. Certain herbs can provide relief without the side effects of conventional painkillers.

- **Turmeric (Curcuma longa):** Turmeric is a powerful anti-inflammatory herb, thanks to its active compound curcumin. It is widely used to reduce pain and inflammation in conditions like arthritis. Turmeric can be taken as a supplement, added to food, or consumed as tea.

- **Willow Bark (Salix alba):** Willow bark is often referred to as nature's aspirin. It contains salicin, which the body converts to salicylic acid, providing pain relief. It is effective for headaches, muscle pain, and arthritis. Willow bark can be taken as a tea or in capsule form.

- **Devil's Claw (Harpagophytum procumbens):** Devil's Claw is known for its analgesic and anti-inflammatory properties, making it effective for treating joint pain, back pain, and arthritis. It can be consumed as a supplement or tea.

- **Boswellia (Boswellia serrata):** Also known as Indian frankincense, Boswellia is an anti-inflammatory herb that helps reduce pain and swelling, particularly in arthritis and inflammatory bowel disease. Boswellia can be taken in capsule form or as a resin extract.

5. Herbs for Skin Health

Herbs can be beneficial for maintaining healthy skin and treating various skin conditions.

- **Calendula (Calendula officinalis):** Calendula is known for its healing and anti-inflammatory properties. It is commonly used to treat cuts, burns, and skin irritations. Calendula can be applied topically as a cream, ointment, or infused oil.

- **Aloe Vera (Aloe barbadensis miller):** Aloe vera is widely used for its soothing and moisturizing properties. It is effective for treating burns, sunburn, and dry skin. Aloe vera gel can be applied directly to the skin.

- **Tea Tree (Melaleuca alternifolia):** Tea tree oil has strong antimicrobial and antiseptic properties, making it effective for treating acne, fungal infections, and minor cuts. It should be diluted with a carrier oil before applying to the skin.

- **Chamomile (Matricaria chamomilla):** Chamomile is gentle and soothing, making it ideal for sensitive skin. It can be used to reduce inflammation, calm irritation, and treat conditions like eczema and dermatitis. Chamomile can be used in a cream, oil, or as a compress.

Herbal medicine offers a natural and holistic approach to treating common ailments. By understanding the specific properties and uses of key herbs, individuals can take an active role in managing their health. While herbs are generally safe and effective, it's important to consult with a healthcare provider, especially if you are taking other medications or have underlying health conditions. Incorporating these herbs into your daily routine can lead to improved well-being and a more balanced, healthful life.

How to Prepare and Use Herbal Remedies Safely

Herbal remedies have been used for centuries to promote health and treat various ailments. While they offer natural alternatives to conventional medicine, it's essential to prepare and use them safely to ensure their effectiveness and minimize the risk of side effects. Understanding the correct methods of preparation, dosages, and potential interactions with other medications is crucial for safe and effective use.

1. Understanding Different Forms of Herbal Remedies

Herbal remedies come in various forms, each with its specific preparation methods and uses. Here are some of the most common forms:

- **Teas (Infusions and Decoctions):**

    - *Infusions* are typically used for delicate parts of the herb, such as leaves, flowers, and seeds. To prepare an infusion, pour boiling water over the herbs and let it steep for 10-20 minutes. Strain the liquid and drink as needed. Chamomile, peppermint, and lemon balm are commonly used in infusions.

    - *Decoctions* are used for tougher parts of the herb, such as roots, bark, and seeds. To make a decoction, simmer the herb in water for 20-30 minutes, then strain and use as directed. Ginger, turmeric, and dandelion root are often prepared as decoctions.

- **Tinctures:** Tinctures are concentrated herbal extracts made by soaking herbs in alcohol or vinegar. They are potent and have a long shelf life. To make a tincture, fill a jar with dried or fresh herbs, cover with alcohol (such as vodka) or vinegar, seal tightly, and store in a dark place for 4-6 weeks, shaking daily. Strain the liquid and store it in a dark glass bottle. Tinctures are taken in small doses, usually by dropper, diluted in water.

- **Herbal Oils and Salves:** Herbal oils are made by infusing herbs in a carrier oil, such as olive or coconut oil. The mixture is heated gently to release the herbs' beneficial properties into the oil. Salves are made by mixing herbal oils with beeswax to create a thicker consistency for topical application. Calendula and comfrey are commonly used in herbal oils and salves for skin healing.

- **Herbal Capsules and Powders:** Herbs can be dried, ground into powder, and encapsulated for easy consumption. This method is convenient for herbs with a strong taste or when a precise dosage is required. Turmeric, spirulina, and ashwagandha are often consumed in capsule or powder form.

- **Poultices and Compresses:** A poultice is made by crushing fresh herbs into a paste and applying them directly to the skin to treat injuries, inflammation, or infections. A compress involves soaking a cloth in an herbal infusion or decoction and applying it to the affected area. Comfrey and plantain are commonly used in poultices.

2. Guidelines for Safe Preparation

When preparing herbal remedies, following safety guidelines is crucial to ensure their efficacy and avoid contamination or spoilage.

- **Use High-Quality Herbs:** Always source herbs from reputable suppliers to ensure they are free from pesticides, contaminants, and adulterants. Fresh, organic herbs are preferable for making remedies.

- **Correct Dosage and Potency:** Use the correct amount of herb for the desired effect. Overuse or incorrect dosages can lead to adverse reactions. Follow recommended guidelines or consult a healthcare professional for specific dosages.

- **Cleanliness and Sterility:** Ensure that all utensils, jars, and storage containers are clean and dry to prevent contamination. Sterilize jars and bottles used for tinctures and oils to prolong shelf life and reduce the risk of mold or bacteria growth.

- **Proper Storage:** Store herbal remedies in dark, airtight containers to protect them from light, heat, and moisture, which can degrade their potency. Label containers with the herb's name and preparation date, and check regularly for signs of spoilage.

- **Avoid Metal Utensils:** When preparing herbal teas or tinctures, avoid using metal utensils, as they can react with certain herbs and affect the remedy's effectiveness. Use wooden, glass, or ceramic tools instead.

3. Safe Usage Practices

Using herbal remedies safely involves understanding their effects, interactions, and any potential side effects.

- **Start with Small Doses:** If you are new to a particular herb, start with a small dose to gauge your body's reaction. Gradually increase the dosage if necessary, while monitoring for any adverse effects.

- **Be Aware of Allergies and Sensitivities:** Some individuals may have allergic reactions or sensitivities to certain herbs. If you experience symptoms such as itching, rash, or gastrointestinal discomfort, discontinue use and consult a healthcare provider.

- **Consider Drug Interactions:** Herbal remedies can interact with prescription medications, leading to reduced efficacy or increased side effects. Consult with a healthcare provider before using herbs, especially if you are taking other medications or have underlying health conditions.

- **Follow Duration Guidelines:** Some herbs are safe for long-term use, while others should be used for short periods. For example, herbs like ashwagandha can be used long-term, while others like echinacea are recommended for short-term use only. Adhere to guidelines for safe usage duration.

- **Pregnancy and Breastfeeding:** Certain herbs are not safe for use during pregnancy or breastfeeding. Always consult with a healthcare provider before using herbal remedies during these periods.

4. Ethical and Sustainable Sourcing

Ethical considerations are also important in herbal medicine. Overharvesting and unsustainable practices can lead to the depletion of valuable plant species.

- **Choose Sustainably Sourced Herbs:** Support companies that prioritize sustainable harvesting practices and fair trade. Look for certifications or information on ethical sourcing when purchasing herbs.

- **Grow Your Own Herbs:** Growing your own herbs is a sustainable option that ensures a fresh supply and reduces reliance on commercially harvested plants. Herbs like mint, basil, and rosemary are easy to grow in home gardens.

- **Respect Traditional Knowledge:** Many herbs have been used for centuries in traditional medicine systems, such as Ayurveda and Traditional Chinese Medicine. Respect and acknowledge the cultural heritage and knowledge of these practices.

Herbal remedies offer a powerful and natural way to support health and well-being, but they must be prepared and used safely. By understanding the various forms of herbal remedies, following proper preparation techniques, and adhering to safe usage practices, you can harness the healing power of herbs effectively. Always consult with a healthcare provider if you have any concerns or are new to herbal medicine, and ensure that your practices are sustainable and respectful of traditional knowledge.

Chapter 12: Nutrition and Meal Planning

Developing a Balanced Meal Plan

Creating a balanced meal plan is essential for maintaining optimal health and well-being. A well-structured plan ensures that your body receives the necessary nutrients in the right proportions to support energy levels, immune function, cognitive health, and overall vitality. A balanced diet is not just about counting calories; it's about nourishing your body with a variety of nutrient-dense foods that promote long-term health.

1. Understanding the Components of a Balanced Diet

A balanced diet includes a variety of foods that provide the necessary macronutrients and micronutrients. The key components include:

- **Macronutrients:**

    o *Carbohydrates:* The primary source of energy for the body. Include complex carbohydrates like whole grains, fruits, and vegetables for sustained energy and fiber.

    o *Proteins:* Essential for muscle repair, hormone production, and immune function. Incorporate a mix of plant-based proteins (like legumes, nuts, and seeds) and animal-based proteins (such as lean meats, fish, eggs, and dairy).

    o *Fats:* Necessary for brain health, hormone production, and the absorption of fat-soluble vitamins. Focus on healthy fats from sources like avocados, nuts, seeds, olive oil, and fatty fish.

- **Micronutrients:**

- *Vitamins and Minerals:* Vital for various bodily functions, including immune support, bone health, and energy production. Ensure a colorful plate with a variety of fruits and vegetables to cover a broad spectrum of vitamins and minerals.

- **Fiber:**

  - Important for digestive health and helps regulate blood sugar levels. Incorporate fiber-rich foods like whole grains, vegetables, fruits, and legumes.

- **Hydration:**

  - Adequate water intake is crucial for overall health, aiding in digestion, circulation, and temperature regulation. Aim to drink at least 8 glasses of water a day, adjusting based on activity level and climate.

2. Steps to Develop a Balanced Meal Plan

Creating a balanced meal plan involves careful planning and consideration of your dietary needs, lifestyle, and health goals.

- **Assess Your Nutritional Needs:**

  - Determine your daily caloric and nutritional requirements based on factors like age, gender, activity level, and health goals. Tools like the MyPlate guide or consultation with a nutritionist can help tailor your plan.

- **Plan Your Meals Around Whole Foods:**

  - Prioritize whole, minimally processed foods. Include a variety of fruits, vegetables, whole grains, lean proteins, and healthy fats in your daily meals. This approach ensures you get the most nutrients and avoid added sugars, unhealthy fats, and preservatives found in processed foods.

- **Balance Macronutrients in Every Meal:**

  - Aim to include a source of protein, healthy fat, and complex carbohydrates in each meal. For example, a balanced breakfast could include eggs (protein), avocado (healthy fat), and whole-grain toast (complex carbohydrates).

- **Incorporate a Variety of Foods:**

  - Variety is key to ensuring you get a wide range of nutrients. Rotate your protein sources (e.g., chicken, fish, beans), vary your fruits and vegetables (aim for different colors), and experiment with whole grains (like quinoa, brown rice, and oats).

- **Plan for Portion Control:**

  - Practice portion control to avoid overeating. Use tools like smaller plates or pre-portioned containers to help manage serving sizes. Focus on eating until you're satisfied, not overly full.

- **Include Snacks Wisely:**

  - Healthy snacks can help maintain energy levels throughout the day. Choose snacks that combine protein and fiber, like Greek yogurt with berries, or hummus with carrot sticks, to keep you satisfied between meals.

- **Plan for Flexibility:**

  - Life can be unpredictable, so plan meals that are easy to prepare and adaptable. Have quick, healthy options available, like frozen vegetables or canned beans, for days when time is limited.

3. Sample Balanced Meal Plan

Here's a sample meal plan to illustrate how to incorporate these principles:

- **Breakfast:**

  - *Oatmeal with Fresh Berries, Nuts, and a Dollop of Greek Yogurt*

    - Whole grains provide sustained energy, berries add vitamins and antioxidants, nuts offer healthy fats and protein, and yogurt contributes probiotics and additional protein.

- **Lunch:**

- o *Grilled Chicken Salad with Mixed Greens, Avocado, Cherry Tomatoes, and a Vinaigrette Dressing*
    - The salad provides a balance of lean protein, healthy fats, and a variety of vitamins and minerals. Use olive oil and vinegar dressing for added healthy fats and flavor.

- **Dinner:**
    - o *Baked Salmon with Quinoa, Steamed Broccoli, and a Side of Sweet Potatoes*
        - Salmon is rich in omega-3 fatty acids, quinoa offers complete protein and fiber, broccoli adds vitamins and minerals, and sweet potatoes provide complex carbohydrates and fiber.

- **Snacks:**
    - o *Apple Slices with Almond Butter*
        - Combines fiber and healthy fats for a satisfying, nutrient-dense snack.
    - o *Carrot Sticks with Hummus*
        - Offers fiber, vitamins, and protein from the chickpeas in hummus.

4. Adapting the Plan for Different Life Stages and Needs

Different life stages and individual needs require adjustments to your meal plan:

- **Children and Adolescents:**
    - o Focus on growth-supporting nutrients like calcium, iron, and protein. Include dairy or fortified plant-based alternatives, lean meats, and plenty of fruits and vegetables.

- **Adults:**

- Prioritize maintaining energy levels and preventing chronic diseases. Emphasize balanced meals with whole grains, lean proteins, healthy fats, and a variety of fruits and vegetables.

- **Seniors:**

  - Focus on nutrient-dense foods that are easy to digest and support bone and joint health. Include calcium-rich foods, fiber, and plenty of hydration. Adjust portion sizes as metabolism slows down.

- **Athletes and Active Individuals:**

  - Increased activity levels may require higher caloric intake, with a focus on protein for muscle repair and carbohydrates for energy. Incorporate post-workout snacks like a protein shake with fruit.

- **Individuals with Specific Health Conditions:**

  - Tailor the meal plan to address specific health needs, such as a low-sodium diet for hypertension, or gluten-free options for those with celiac disease. Always consult with a healthcare provider for personalized guidance.

5. Maintaining Long-Term Success

Developing a balanced meal plan is just the beginning. To ensure long-term success:

- **Regularly Reevaluate Your Plan:**

  - Your dietary needs can change due to age, health conditions, or lifestyle shifts. Reassess your meal plan periodically to ensure it still meets your nutritional needs.

- **Stay Informed:**

  - Keep up with the latest nutrition research and recommendations. Understanding the science behind your food choices can motivate you to maintain healthy habits.

- **Seek Support:**

- Whether through a nutritionist, a support group, or a community, finding like-minded individuals can help you stay committed to your balanced meal plan.

- **Allow for Flexibility and Enjoyment:**

  - A balanced diet doesn't mean depriving yourself. Allow occasional indulgences and focus on overall patterns rather than perfection. Enjoy your meals and appreciate the nourishment they provide.

Developing a balanced meal plan is a cornerstone of sustainable health. By understanding the components of a balanced diet, planning your meals thoughtfully, and making adjustments based on your specific needs, you can create a nutrition plan that supports long-term wellness. Remember, balance is not just about what you eat, but also about how you approach food and nourishment in your life.

Recipes for Health and Vitality

Creating delicious, nutrient-dense recipes is a powerful way to support your health and vitality. These recipes focus on whole, natural ingredients that provide essential vitamins, minerals, and antioxidants to fuel your body and mind. Below are some easy-to-prepare, balanced recipes that cater to various dietary preferences and promote overall well-being.

1. Green Smoothie Bowl

A vibrant and refreshing smoothie bowl that's packed with vitamins, minerals, and fiber. It's an excellent way to start your day or enjoy as a post-workout meal.

Ingredients:

- 1 cup spinach or kale leaves

- 1 frozen banana

- ½ cup frozen berries (blueberries or strawberries)

- ½ avocado

- 1 tablespoon chia seeds or flaxseeds

- 1 tablespoon almond butter or peanut butter

- 1 cup unsweetened almond milk or coconut water

- Optional toppings: sliced banana, fresh berries, granola, coconut flakes, nuts

Instructions:

1. In a blender, combine spinach or kale, frozen banana, frozen berries, avocado, chia seeds, almond butter, and almond milk.

2. Blend until smooth and creamy. Adjust the consistency with more almond milk if needed.

3. Pour the smoothie into a bowl and add your favorite toppings like sliced banana, fresh berries, granola, and coconut flakes.

4. Enjoy immediately as a nourishing breakfast or snack.

2. Quinoa and Roasted Vegetable Salad

A satisfying and nutrient-packed salad that's perfect for lunch or dinner. Quinoa is a complete protein, making this dish not only delicious but also filling and nourishing.

Ingredients:

- 1 cup quinoa, rinsed

- 2 cups water or vegetable broth

- 1 red bell pepper, diced

- 1 zucchini, sliced

- 1 carrot, sliced

- 1 red onion, sliced

- 2 tablespoons olive oil

- Salt and pepper to taste

- 1 teaspoon dried oregano or thyme

- 1 cup cherry tomatoes, halved

- 1 cup baby spinach or arugula

- ¼ cup feta cheese or goat cheese (optional)

- Fresh lemon juice and olive oil for dressing

Instructions:

1. Preheat your oven to 400°F (200°C). Line a baking sheet with parchment paper.

2. Cook the quinoa by combining it with water or broth in a pot. Bring to a boil, then reduce the heat, cover, and simmer for about 15 minutes until the liquid is absorbed and the quinoa is fluffy. Set aside to cool.

3. Meanwhile, toss the diced red pepper, zucchini, carrot, and red onion with olive oil, salt, pepper, and oregano. Spread them on the baking sheet and roast in the oven for 20-25 minutes until they are tender and slightly caramelized.

4. In a large mixing bowl, combine the cooked quinoa, roasted vegetables, cherry tomatoes, and baby spinach.

5. If using, crumble feta or goat cheese on top.

6. Drizzle with fresh lemon juice and a bit of olive oil before serving.

3. Turmeric and Ginger Immune-Boosting Soup

This warming soup is infused with anti-inflammatory spices like turmeric and ginger, perfect for supporting your immune system and promoting overall vitality.

Ingredients:

- 1 tablespoon olive oil or coconut oil

- 1 onion, diced

- 3 cloves garlic, minced

- 1 tablespoon fresh ginger, grated

- 1 tablespoon turmeric powder

- 1 teaspoon ground cumin

- 1 teaspoon ground coriander

- 1 large carrot, diced

- 1 sweet potato, peeled and diced

- 4 cups vegetable broth or water

- 1 can (14 oz) coconut milk

- Salt and pepper to taste

- 1 cup kale or spinach, chopped

- Fresh cilantro or parsley for garnish

- Fresh lemon juice for serving

Instructions:

1. In a large pot, heat the olive oil over medium heat. Add the onion and sauté until softened, about 5 minutes.

2. Stir in the garlic, ginger, turmeric, cumin, and coriander, and cook for another minute until fragrant.

3. Add the diced carrot and sweet potato, and stir to coat with the spices.

4. Pour in the vegetable broth or water and bring to a boil. Reduce the heat and simmer for 15-20 minutes until the vegetables are tender.

5. Stir in the coconut milk and chopped kale or spinach. Simmer for an additional 5 minutes.

6. Season with salt and pepper to taste.

7. Serve the soup hot, garnished with fresh cilantro or parsley, and a squeeze of lemon juice for added brightness.

4. Baked Salmon with Garlic and Herbs

Salmon is rich in omega-3 fatty acids, which are crucial for brain health and reducing inflammation. This simple yet flavorful dish is perfect for a quick and nutritious dinner.

Ingredients:

- 4 salmon fillets (about 6 oz each)
- 2 tablespoons olive oil
- 3 cloves garlic, minced
- 1 teaspoon dried oregano
- 1 teaspoon dried thyme
- 1 teaspoon dried basil
- Salt and pepper to taste
- Fresh lemon slices and fresh herbs (like parsley or dill) for garnish

Instructions:

1. Preheat your oven to 400°F (200°C). Line a baking sheet with foil or parchment paper.
2. In a small bowl, mix together the olive oil, minced garlic, oregano, thyme, basil, salt, and pepper.
3. Place the salmon fillets on the prepared baking sheet. Brush the garlic and herb mixture evenly over the top of each fillet.
4. Place lemon slices on top of the salmon.
5. Bake for 12-15 minutes, or until the salmon is cooked through and flakes easily with a fork.

6. Garnish with fresh herbs and serve with a side of steamed vegetables or a fresh green salad.

5. Overnight Chia Pudding

This easy-to-make chia pudding is a perfect breakfast or snack that's high in fiber, omega-3 fatty acids, and protein. Customize it with your favorite toppings for a delicious and nutritious treat.

Ingredients:

- 3 tablespoons chia seeds
- 1 cup unsweetened almond milk or coconut milk
- 1 tablespoon maple syrup or honey
- ½ teaspoon vanilla extract
- Optional toppings: fresh berries, sliced banana, nuts, seeds, coconut flakes, dark chocolate shavings

Instructions:

1. In a mixing bowl, whisk together the chia seeds, almond milk, maple syrup, and vanilla extract.
2. Let the mixture sit for 5 minutes, then whisk again to prevent clumping.
3. Cover the bowl and refrigerate for at least 4 hours or overnight, until the chia seeds have absorbed the liquid and the pudding has thickened.
4. Before serving, stir the pudding well and add your favorite toppings like fresh berries, nuts, or coconut flakes.
5. Enjoy as a nutritious breakfast, snack, or even a healthy dessert.

These recipes are designed to provide you with the nutrients and energy needed to support your health and vitality. By incorporating a variety of whole foods, healthy fats, lean proteins, and plenty of fruits and vegetables, you can create meals that are not only delicious but also deeply nourishing for your body and mind. Experiment with these recipes, adjust them to suit your tastes and dietary needs, and enjoy the process of cooking and eating foods that truly support your well-being.

Adapting Your Diet for Different Life Stages and Needs

As we journey through different stages of life, our nutritional needs evolve, requiring adjustments to our diet to support optimal health and well-being. From childhood to old age, each life stage has unique demands that can be met through thoughtful dietary choices. Understanding these needs and how to adapt your diet accordingly is crucial for maintaining vitality, preventing illness, and promoting longevity.

1. Childhood and Adolescence

Nutritional Needs:

- **Growth and Development:** During these stages, the body requires a higher intake of calories, protein, and essential nutrients like calcium, iron, and vitamins to support rapid growth and development.

- **Cognitive Function:** Nutrients like omega-3 fatty acids, found in fish, flaxseeds, and walnuts, are vital for brain development and cognitive function.

Dietary Recommendations:

- **Balanced Diet:** Focus on a diet rich in whole foods, including fruits, vegetables, whole grains, lean proteins, and healthy fats.

- **Calcium and Vitamin D:** Ensure adequate intake of calcium-rich foods (e.g., dairy, leafy greens) and vitamin D (from sunlight and fortified foods) to support bone health.

- **Limit Processed Foods:** Minimize the consumption of sugary snacks, sodas, and highly processed foods that can lead to obesity and other health issues.

2. Adulthood

Nutritional Needs:

- **Maintenance and Prevention:** The focus shifts to maintaining health, preventing chronic diseases, and managing energy levels.

- **Metabolism:** Metabolic rate may slow down, necessitating a balanced intake of calories to prevent weight gain.

Dietary Recommendations:

- **Diverse Nutrients:** Include a wide variety of nutrient-dense foods to ensure a broad intake of vitamins, minerals, and antioxidants.

- **Healthy Fats:** Incorporate sources of healthy fats, such as avocados, nuts, seeds, and olive oil, to support heart health.

- **Fiber-Rich Foods:** Consume plenty of fiber from fruits, vegetables, and whole grains to promote digestive health and prevent conditions like heart disease and diabetes.

3. Pregnancy and Lactation

Nutritional Needs:

- **Increased Nutrient Requirements:** Pregnant and lactating women need additional nutrients like folic acid, iron, calcium, and omega-3 fatty acids to support the growth and development of the baby and maintain their own health.

Dietary Recommendations:

- **Folic Acid:** Ensure adequate intake of folic acid through leafy greens, legumes, and fortified grains to prevent neural tube defects.

- **Iron-Rich Foods:** Consume iron-rich foods like lean meats, beans, and spinach to support increased blood volume and prevent anemia.

- **Hydration:** Stay well-hydrated, especially during lactation, to support milk production and overall well-being.

4. Midlife

Nutritional Needs:

- **Hormonal Changes:** For women, menopause brings hormonal changes that can affect metabolism, bone density, and heart health. Men may also experience changes in muscle mass and energy levels.

Dietary Recommendations:

- **Bone Health:** Increase intake of calcium and vitamin D to support bone health and prevent osteoporosis.

- **Phytoestrogens:** Incorporate foods like soy, flaxseeds, and whole grains that contain phytoestrogens, which may help balance hormone levels during menopause.

- **Heart Health:** Focus on heart-healthy foods like fatty fish, nuts, and seeds, and reduce saturated fats and refined sugars to protect cardiovascular health.

5. Older Adulthood

Nutritional Needs:

- **Nutrient Absorption:** As we age, the body's ability to absorb certain nutrients, such as vitamin B12 and calcium, may decrease.

- **Muscle Mass and Strength:** Maintaining muscle mass and strength becomes important for mobility and independence.

Dietary Recommendations:

- **Nutrient-Dense Foods:** Prioritize nutrient-dense foods that provide essential vitamins and minerals without excessive calories.

- **Protein:** Ensure sufficient protein intake to preserve muscle mass and support overall health. Sources include lean meats, fish, beans, and dairy.

- **Hydration:** Older adults may experience a diminished sense of thirst, so it's important to consciously stay hydrated by drinking water regularly and including hydrating foods like fruits and vegetables.

6. Special Dietary Needs

Chronic Conditions: Individuals with chronic conditions like diabetes, heart disease, or digestive disorders may need to follow specific dietary guidelines to manage their condition.

- **Personalized Nutrition:** Work with a healthcare provider or nutritionist to develop a personalized diet plan that addresses individual health concerns and promotes overall well-being.

Active Lifestyles: Athletes and those with physically demanding jobs require higher caloric intake and increased protein to support energy levels, muscle repair, and recovery.

- **Balanced Intake:** Focus on a balanced intake of carbohydrates for energy, protein for muscle repair, and fats for sustained energy.

Adapting your diet to align with the different stages of life and your unique needs is essential for maintaining health, preventing disease, and promoting longevity. By making thoughtful, informed choices, you can ensure that your diet provides the right balance of nutrients to support your body's changing requirements, helping you to live a vibrant, healthy life at every stage.

PART THREE:

ADVANCED TOPICS

Chapter 13: Functional Medicine and Holistic Health

The Role of Functional Medicine in Modern Healthcare

Functional medicine represents a paradigm shift in how we approach healthcare, moving away from traditional, symptom-focused treatments toward a more holistic, patient-centered model. By addressing the root causes of disease rather than merely treating symptoms, functional medicine offers a comprehensive and personalized approach that is increasingly being recognized for its potential to transform modern healthcare.

1. Understanding Functional Medicine

Functional medicine is an integrative approach that combines the best of conventional medicine with evidence-based alternative therapies. It focuses on understanding the complex interactions between genetics, environment, and lifestyle factors that influence long-term health and chronic disease.

Core Principles:

- **Personalized Care:** Each patient is unique, and functional medicine tailors treatment plans to the individual's specific genetic makeup, environmental exposures, and lifestyle choices.

- **Root Cause Focus:** Rather than just addressing symptoms, functional medicine seeks to identify and treat the underlying causes of illness.

- **Patient-Centered:** The patient is seen as a whole person, with their physical, emotional, mental, and spiritual health all taken into consideration.

2. The Shift from Conventional to Functional Medicine

Conventional medicine, while effective for acute care and emergency situations, often falls short in managing chronic conditions like diabetes, heart disease, and autoimmune disorders. These diseases are complex and multifactorial, often requiring more than just medication to manage.

Key Differences:

- **Symptom Management vs. Root Cause:** Traditional medicine often focuses on managing symptoms through medication or surgery, whereas functional medicine aims to uncover and address the root causes, such as inflammation, nutritional deficiencies, or hormonal imbalances.

- **Standardized vs. Personalized Treatment:** Conventional approaches often involve standardized treatment protocols, while functional medicine emphasizes personalized care based on a deep understanding of the individual.

- **Reactive vs. Proactive:** Traditional healthcare can be reactive, addressing issues as they arise, whereas functional medicine emphasizes prevention and proactive health management through lifestyle changes.

3. Integrating Functional Medicine into Modern Healthcare

Integrating functional medicine into the broader healthcare system involves a collaborative approach where functional medicine practitioners work alongside conventional healthcare providers. This integration can offer a more comprehensive care model that addresses both acute and chronic health issues.

Benefits of Integration:

- **Holistic Health Management:** By combining the strengths of both approaches, patients receive care that addresses the immediate symptoms and the underlying causes of their conditions.

- **Improved Outcomes:** Patients often experience improved outcomes, including better management of chronic conditions, reduced dependence on medications, and enhanced overall well-being.

- **Cost-Effective:** While the initial investment in functional medicine may be higher due to more in-depth testing and personalized treatment plans, it can lead to long-term cost savings by reducing the need for ongoing medical interventions and hospitalizations.

4. Functional Medicine in Chronic Disease Management

Chronic diseases, such as diabetes, heart disease, and autoimmune disorders, are on the rise globally. Functional medicine offers a promising approach to managing these conditions by addressing the lifestyle and environmental factors that contribute to their development.

Key Strategies:

- **Nutrition:** A cornerstone of functional medicine is the use of diet to manage and even reverse chronic conditions. Anti-inflammatory diets, elimination diets, and individualized nutrition plans are common tools.

- **Lifestyle Interventions:** Stress management, sleep optimization, and regular physical activity are integral components of functional medicine, helping to create a foundation for health.

- **Supplements and Botanicals:** Functional medicine often incorporates the use of vitamins, minerals, herbs, and other supplements to support the body's natural healing processes.

5. Case Studies and Success Stories

Many individuals have experienced significant improvements in their health through functional medicine. From reversing type 2 diabetes to managing autoimmune disorders, functional medicine has provided patients with new hope and improved quality of life.

Examples:

- **Autoimmune Disorders:** Patients with conditions like Hashimoto's thyroiditis or rheumatoid arthritis have found relief through functional medicine's focus on reducing inflammation and supporting the immune system.

- **Metabolic Disorders:** Individuals with metabolic syndrome or insulin resistance have successfully managed their conditions through personalized nutrition and lifestyle interventions.

6. The Future of Functional Medicine

As more healthcare providers recognize the benefits of functional medicine, its role in modern healthcare is likely to expand. The focus on prevention, patient empowerment, and holistic care aligns with the growing demand for personalized and integrative healthcare solutions.

Challenges and Opportunities:

- **Education and Training:** As the field grows, there is a need for more education and training opportunities for healthcare providers to learn functional medicine principles.

- **Research and Evidence:** Ongoing research is essential to build a robust evidence base that supports the efficacy of functional medicine approaches.

- **Access and Affordability:** Making functional medicine more accessible and affordable will be key to its widespread adoption.

The role of functional medicine in modern healthcare is increasingly vital as it offers a comprehensive, patient-centered approach to health and wellness. By addressing the root causes of disease and focusing on personalized care, functional medicine has the potential to transform how we manage chronic conditions and promote long-term health. As the healthcare landscape continues to evolve, functional medicine will likely play an integral role in shaping the future of healthcare, offering hope and healing to those seeking a more holistic path to wellness.

Integrating Functional Medicine Principles into Your Life

Integrating functional medicine principles into your daily life is a transformative journey that requires a holistic and personalized approach. Unlike conventional medicine, which often focuses on symptom management, functional medicine delves deeper into the root causes of health issues, emphasizing prevention, individualized care, and a whole-body approach to wellness. This chapter will guide you through practical steps to incorporate these principles into your life, empowering you to take control of your health.

1. Understanding Your Unique Health Profile

The foundation of functional medicine is the recognition that each individual is unique, with specific genetic, environmental, and lifestyle factors influencing their health. The first step in integrating functional medicine principles is to understand your unique health profile.

Key Actions:

- **Genetic Testing:** Consider genetic testing to uncover predispositions to certain health conditions. This information can guide personalized nutrition, exercise, and lifestyle plans.

- **Comprehensive Health Assessment:** Work with a functional medicine practitioner to conduct a thorough health assessment, including detailed medical history, lab tests, and an analysis of your lifestyle, diet, and environment.

- **Personal Health Goals:** Define clear health goals based on your assessment, whether it's improving energy levels, managing a chronic condition, or enhancing overall well-being.

2. Embracing a Whole Foods, Nutrient-Dense Diet

Nutrition is at the core of functional medicine. A whole foods, nutrient-dense diet can help prevent and reverse many chronic conditions by providing the body with the essential nutrients it needs to function optimally.

Key Actions:

- **Eliminate Processed Foods:** Gradually remove processed foods, refined sugars, and unhealthy fats from your diet. These foods can contribute to inflammation, insulin resistance, and other health issues.

- **Focus on Nutrient-Dense Foods:** Incorporate a variety of fruits, vegetables, lean proteins, healthy fats, and whole grains. Organic and locally-sourced foods are ideal to reduce exposure to toxins and maximize nutritional value.

- **Personalized Nutrition Plans:** Tailor your diet to your unique needs, possibly incorporating specific diets like anti-inflammatory, ketogenic, or elimination diets based on your health profile and goals.

3. Prioritizing Gut Health

Gut health is central to functional medicine, as the gut is connected to many aspects of overall health, including immunity, mental health, and chronic disease prevention.

Key Actions:

- **Probiotics and Prebiotics:** Include probiotic-rich foods like yogurt, kefir, and fermented vegetables, and prebiotic foods like garlic, onions, and asparagus, to support a healthy gut microbiome.

- **Identify and Address Food Sensitivities:** Work with your practitioner to identify food sensitivities or intolerances that may be affecting your gut health and overall well-being.

- **Gut-Healing Protocols:** Consider gut-healing protocols that include bone broth, glutamine, and specific supplements to repair the gut lining and reduce inflammation.

4. Balancing Hormones Naturally

Hormonal imbalances can lead to a variety of health issues, from fatigue and weight gain to mood swings and reproductive problems. Functional medicine emphasizes natural approaches to restore hormonal balance.

Key Actions:

- **Stress Management:** Chronic stress can disrupt hormone balance. Incorporate stress-reducing practices like yoga, meditation, deep breathing, and adequate sleep into your daily routine.

- **Nutritional Support:** Ensure your diet includes essential nutrients like magnesium, vitamin D, and omega-3 fatty acids, which are crucial for hormone production and balance.

- **Detoxification:** Reduce exposure to endocrine disruptors found in plastics, pesticides, and personal care products. Support liver detoxification to help your body eliminate these harmful substances.

5. Implementing Regular Physical Activity

Exercise is a powerful tool in functional medicine, offering benefits that range from improved cardiovascular health to enhanced mental clarity and stress reduction.

Key Actions:

- **Personalized Exercise Plan:** Develop a personalized exercise plan that suits your body's needs and your lifestyle. This might include a mix of cardiovascular exercises, strength training, flexibility, and balance exercises.

- **Consistency Over Intensity:** Focus on consistency rather than intensity. Regular moderate exercise, such as daily walking, yoga, or swimming, can have profound health benefits.

- **Movement Throughout the Day:** Integrate movement into your daily routine, such as taking breaks to stretch, using a standing desk, or engaging in short bursts of physical activity.

6. Enhancing Sleep Quality

Sleep is a critical component of functional medicine, as it plays a vital role in healing, recovery, and overall health.

Key Actions:

- **Establish a Sleep Routine:** Create a consistent sleep schedule by going to bed and waking up at the same time every day, even on weekends.

- **Optimize Sleep Environment:** Ensure your sleep environment is conducive to rest, with a comfortable mattress, cool temperature, and minimal light and noise.

- **Address Sleep Disruptors:** Identify and address factors that may disrupt sleep, such as caffeine consumption, late-night screen use, or unresolved stress and anxiety.

7. Supporting Detoxification Pathways

Detoxification is an ongoing process in the body, crucial for eliminating toxins and maintaining health. Functional medicine emphasizes supporting the body's natural detox pathways.

Key Actions:

- **Hydration:** Drink plenty of water to support kidney function and the elimination of toxins through urine.

- **Liver Support:** Incorporate foods like cruciferous vegetables, garlic, and beets, which support liver detoxification. Consider supplements like milk thistle and dandelion root under the guidance of a healthcare provider.

- **Sweating:** Engage in activities that promote sweating, such as exercise or sauna sessions, to help eliminate toxins through the skin.

8. Cultivating a Positive Mindset

A positive mindset is integral to healing and overall wellness. Functional medicine encourages the development of mental and emotional resilience.

Key Actions:

- **Mindfulness and Meditation:** Practice mindfulness and meditation regularly to reduce stress, improve focus, and foster emotional balance.

- **Positive Affirmations:** Use positive affirmations to reframe negative thoughts and cultivate a growth mindset.

- **Community and Relationships:** Surround yourself with supportive and positive relationships, and engage in community activities that foster a sense of belonging and purpose.

9. Empowering Yourself Through Education and Action

Empowerment is a key principle in functional medicine, encouraging individuals to take an active role in their health journey.

Key Actions:

- **Continual Learning:** Educate yourself about your health conditions, functional medicine principles, and the latest research in holistic health.

- **Take Action:** Implement small, manageable changes consistently, building upon them as you progress. This could be as simple as adding more vegetables to your diet or setting aside time for daily exercise.

- **Work with a Practitioner:** Consider working with a functional medicine practitioner who can provide personalized guidance and support your journey towards optimal health.

Integrating functional medicine principles into your life is a journey toward long-term health and wellness. By addressing the root causes of health issues, embracing a whole-body approach, and making personalized lifestyle changes, you can achieve a higher level of well-being. This approach empowers you to take control of your health, leading to a more vibrant, balanced, and fulfilling life.

Case Studies and Success Stories

Case studies and success stories provide compelling evidence of the transformative power of functional medicine. They offer real-life examples of how personalized, root-cause-focused care can lead to significant health improvements, even in cases where conventional medicine has failed to provide relief. In this chapter, we'll explore several case studies and success stories that highlight the effectiveness of functional medicine in addressing chronic health conditions and promoting overall well-being.

Case Study 1: Reversing Type 2 Diabetes

Background:

John, a 52-year-old male, had been struggling with type 2 diabetes for over a decade. Despite being on multiple medications, his blood sugar levels remained poorly controlled, and he experienced frequent episodes of fatigue, neuropathy, and weight gain.

Functional **Medicine** **Approach:**
John's functional medicine practitioner took a comprehensive approach, starting with an in-depth evaluation of his lifestyle, diet, and medical history. Key interventions included:

- **Dietary Changes:** John was placed on a low-carbohydrate, high-fat (LCHF) diet, focusing on whole foods, healthy fats, and plenty of non-starchy vegetables. He eliminated processed foods, refined sugars, and grains from his diet.

- **Exercise:** A personalized exercise plan was created, incorporating both aerobic exercise and resistance training to improve insulin sensitivity.

- **Gut Health:** John's gut health was assessed, and he was found to have an imbalance in his gut microbiome. A regimen of probiotics and prebiotics was introduced to restore balance, along with a protocol to reduce inflammation.

- **Stress Management:** Mindfulness practices and stress reduction techniques were implemented to lower cortisol levels, which can negatively impact blood sugar control.

Results:

Within six months, John experienced significant improvements. His HbA1c levels dropped from 8.5% to 6.2%, indicating much better blood sugar control. He lost 30 pounds, his energy levels improved, and the symptoms of neuropathy began to fade. By the end of the year, John was able to reduce his medication under his doctor's supervision, and he felt empowered to maintain his health through the lifestyle changes he had adopted.

Case Study 2: Overcoming Chronic Fatigue Syndrome

Background:

Sarah, a 38-year-old woman, had been suffering from chronic fatigue syndrome (CFS) for several years. She experienced overwhelming fatigue, brain fog, and muscle pain, which severely impacted her quality of life. Conventional treatments had offered little relief, and she was becoming increasingly frustrated and hopeless.

Functional   **Medicine**   **Approach:**

Sarah's functional medicine practitioner conducted extensive testing, revealing several underlying issues, including adrenal fatigue, gut dysbiosis, and heavy metal toxicity. The treatment plan included:

- **Adrenal Support:** Sarah was given adaptogenic herbs like ashwagandha and rhodiola to support adrenal function and reduce stress. She also adopted a consistent sleep schedule and prioritized rest and relaxation.

- **Gut Healing:** A gut-healing protocol was introduced, including the elimination of food sensitivities, supplementation with digestive enzymes, and the use of a high-potency probiotic.

- **Detoxification:** A gentle detoxification program was implemented to address heavy metal toxicity, using chelating agents and liver-supportive herbs like milk thistle.

- **Nutritional Support:** Sarah's diet was modified to include nutrient-dense, anti-inflammatory foods, with a focus on high-quality proteins, healthy fats, and antioxidant-rich vegetables.

Results:

Over the course of a year, Sarah's symptoms gradually improved. Her energy levels increased, brain fog diminished, and she was able to resume activities she had previously given up due to fatigue. By the end of the treatment, Sarah reported feeling like she had regained control of her life and was no longer defined by her illness.

Case Study 3: Healing Autoimmune Disease

Background:

Michael, a 45-year-old male, was diagnosed with Hashimoto's thyroiditis, an autoimmune thyroid disorder. He experienced symptoms like fatigue, weight gain, hair loss, and depression. Despite being on thyroid medication, his symptoms persisted, and he was concerned about the long-term effects of his condition.

Functional   Medicine   Approach:

Michael's functional medicine practitioner focused on identifying and addressing the root causes of his autoimmune condition. The treatment plan included:

- **Gluten-Free Diet:** Given the strong connection between gluten and autoimmune thyroid disorders, Michael was advised to adopt a strict gluten-free diet, which also eliminated other common allergens like dairy and soy.

- **Immune System Modulation:** Supplements like vitamin D, omega-3 fatty acids, and curcumin were used to modulate the immune response and reduce inflammation.

- **Gut Health Restoration:** Michael underwent a gut-healing protocol to address leaky gut syndrome, which involved eliminating trigger foods, taking gut-healing supplements, and using probiotics.

- **Stress Reduction:** Stress management techniques, including meditation, yoga, and time in nature, were integrated into Michael's daily routine to help lower cortisol levels and support immune function.

Results:

After nine months, Michael experienced a significant reduction in symptoms. His energy levels improved, his weight stabilized, and he noticed less hair loss. Lab tests showed a decrease in thyroid antibodies, indicating a reduction in the autoimmune attack on his thyroid. Michael felt more empowered and educated about managing his condition and was able to reduce his medication dosage under his doctor's guidance.

Success Story: A Holistic Approach to Mental Health

Background:

Emma, a 29-year-old woman, had been dealing with anxiety and depression for several years. She had tried various medications and therapies with limited success and was looking for a more holistic approach to mental health.

Functional   Medicine   Approach:

Emma's functional medicine practitioner took a comprehensive approach, focusing on the mind-body connection and the role of nutrition and lifestyle in mental health. The treatment plan included:

- **Nutritional Therapy:** Emma's diet was optimized to include foods rich in omega-3 fatty acids, B vitamins, and magnesium, which are crucial for brain health. She also reduced her intake of sugar and processed foods.

- **Hormonal Balance:** Hormonal imbalances were addressed through the use of herbal supplements and lifestyle modifications, including stress management and sleep optimization.

- **Mindfulness and Meditation:** Emma was introduced to mindfulness practices and meditation, which she incorporated into her daily routine to help manage anxiety and improve emotional resilience.

- **Exercise:** Regular physical activity, including yoga and outdoor walks, was encouraged to boost endorphins and improve mood.

Results:

Over the course of six months, Emma experienced a significant improvement in her mental health. Her anxiety levels decreased, and she reported feeling more emotionally balanced and resilient. She was able to taper off her medication under the guidance of her healthcare provider and felt more empowered to maintain her mental health through the lifestyle changes she had adopted.

These case studies and success stories demonstrate the profound impact that functional medicine can have on individuals facing chronic health challenges. By addressing the root causes of illness and taking a personalized, holistic approach to care, functional medicine offers hope and healing to those who may have struggled to find relief through conventional means. These stories are not just about overcoming illness; they are about reclaiming health, vitality, and the confidence to live life to the fullest.

Chapter 14: Preventing and Reversing Chronic Illness

Understanding the Root Causes of Chronic Diseases

Chronic diseases, such as diabetes, heart disease, cancer, and autoimmune disorders, are among the leading causes of death and disability worldwide. While conventional medicine often focuses on managing symptoms, functional medicine emphasizes understanding and addressing the root causes of these conditions. This approach is essential for effective prevention, treatment, and long-term health management.

The Complexity of Chronic Diseases

Chronic diseases are rarely caused by a single factor; they are usually the result of a complex interplay of genetic, environmental, and lifestyle factors. This complexity means that a one-size-fits-all approach is often insufficient. Instead, identifying and addressing the unique combination of factors contributing to an individual's condition is key to achieving lasting health improvements.

Key Root Causes of Chronic Diseases

1. **Inflammation:**

   o Chronic inflammation is a common underlying factor in many chronic diseases. It can result from poor diet, stress, environmental toxins, infections, or a sedentary lifestyle. Over time, inflammation can damage tissues and organs, leading to conditions like heart disease, arthritis, and cancer.

2. **Oxidative Stress:**

- Oxidative stress occurs when there is an imbalance between free radicals and antioxidants in the body. Free radicals can cause cellular damage, contributing to aging and chronic diseases such as Alzheimer's, Parkinson's, and cardiovascular diseases.

3. **Insulin Resistance:**

   - Insulin resistance, where cells in the body become less responsive to insulin, is a key factor in the development of type 2 diabetes, obesity, and metabolic syndrome. This condition is often driven by poor diet, lack of exercise, and chronic stress.

4. **Gut Dysbiosis:**

   - The health of the gut microbiome plays a crucial role in overall health. An imbalance in the gut flora, known as gut dysbiosis, can contribute to chronic diseases such as inflammatory bowel disease (IBD), autoimmune disorders, and even mental health conditions like depression and anxiety.

5. **Hormonal Imbalances:**

   - Hormones regulate many of the body's processes, including metabolism, mood, and immune function. Imbalances in hormones such as cortisol, thyroid hormones, and sex hormones can contribute to conditions like hypothyroidism, adrenal fatigue, and polycystic ovary syndrome (PCOS).

6. **Toxicity:**

   - Exposure to environmental toxins, such as heavy metals, pesticides, and pollutants, can overwhelm the body's detoxification systems, leading to chronic diseases. Toxins can accumulate in the body, contributing to conditions like cancer, neurological disorders, and chronic fatigue syndrome.

7. **Nutrient Deficiencies:**

   - A lack of essential nutrients, such as vitamins, minerals, and essential fatty acids, can impair bodily functions and lead to chronic diseases. For example, vitamin D deficiency has been linked to osteoporosis, autoimmune diseases, and certain cancers.

8. **Chronic Stress:**

   o Chronic stress can have a profound impact on health, leading to conditions such as hypertension, anxiety, depression, and immune dysfunction. The stress response triggers the release of hormones like cortisol, which can have damaging effects when elevated over long periods.

Functional Medicine's Approach to Root Causes

Functional medicine practitioners aim to identify and address these root causes through a comprehensive, individualized approach. This involves:

- **Detailed Patient History:** Understanding the patient's health history, lifestyle, diet, and environmental exposures.

- **Advanced Testing:** Using functional lab tests to assess inflammation, gut health, nutrient status, hormone levels, and toxin exposure.

- **Personalized Treatment Plans:** Developing treatment plans that include dietary changes, stress management techniques, detoxification protocols, and targeted supplementation to address the root causes of disease.

The Importance of Addressing Root Causes

By focusing on the root causes rather than just the symptoms, functional medicine can help patients achieve more effective and sustainable health outcomes. This approach not only improves symptoms but also reduces the risk of future chronic diseases, leading to a higher quality of life and longevity.

Strategies for Prevention and Reversal

Preventing and reversing chronic diseases is not only possible but essential for living a long and healthy life. While genetics play a role, lifestyle and environmental factors are often the primary drivers of chronic conditions. By adopting evidence-based strategies, individuals can significantly reduce their risk of developing chronic diseases and, in some cases, even reverse existing conditions.

1. Embrace a Nutrient-Dense Diet

A balanced, nutrient-rich diet is foundational for both preventing and reversing chronic diseases. This includes:

- **Whole Foods:** Focus on whole, unprocessed foods that are rich in vitamins, minerals, antioxidants, and fiber. Vegetables, fruits, lean proteins, healthy fats, and whole grains should form the basis of your diet.

- **Anti-Inflammatory Foods:** Incorporate foods that fight inflammation, such as fatty fish (rich in omega-3 fatty acids), turmeric, berries, leafy greens, and nuts.

- **Limit Sugar and Refined Carbohydrates:** High sugar intake is linked to obesity, insulin resistance, and type 2 diabetes. Reducing or eliminating refined sugars and processed foods can improve blood sugar control and reduce inflammation.

- **Avoid Trans Fats:** Trans fats are harmful to heart health and are found in many processed foods. Opt for healthy fats like olive oil, avocados, and nuts instead.

2. Maintain a Healthy Weight

Obesity is a significant risk factor for many chronic diseases, including heart disease, diabetes, and certain cancers. Achieving and maintaining a healthy weight through diet and exercise is crucial for prevention and reversal. Strategies include:

- **Portion Control:** Be mindful of portion sizes to avoid overeating, especially high-calorie foods.

- **Regular Physical Activity:** Engage in regular exercise to burn calories and improve overall health.

- **Balanced Macronutrient Intake:** Ensure your diet has the right balance of carbohydrates, proteins, and fats to support your metabolism and energy needs.

3. Engage in Regular Physical Activity

Physical activity is one of the most effective ways to prevent and reverse chronic diseases. Benefits include:

- **Improved Cardiovascular Health:** Exercise strengthens the heart and improves circulation, reducing the risk of heart disease and stroke.

- **Enhanced Insulin Sensitivity:** Regular exercise helps regulate blood sugar levels and can prevent or reverse type 2 diabetes.

- **Weight Management:** Physical activity helps maintain a healthy weight and prevents obesity-related diseases.

- **Mental Health Benefits:** Exercise reduces stress, anxiety, and depression, all of which can negatively impact physical health.

4. Manage Stress Effectively

Chronic stress is a contributing factor to many chronic diseases. Long-term stress can lead to hypertension, heart disease, and immune system dysfunction. Strategies to manage stress include:

- **Mindfulness and Meditation:** Practices like meditation, deep breathing exercises, and yoga can help calm the mind and reduce stress levels.

- **Time Management:** Organizing your time effectively can reduce the feeling of being overwhelmed and stressed.

- **Hobbies and Leisure Activities:** Engaging in activities you enjoy can provide a mental break from stress and promote relaxation.

5. Prioritize Sleep

Sleep is essential for the body's repair and recovery processes. Poor sleep quality or insufficient sleep is linked to an increased risk of obesity, diabetes, cardiovascular disease, and weakened immune function. To improve sleep:

- **Establish a Regular Sleep Schedule:** Go to bed and wake up at the same time each day to regulate your body's internal clock.

- **Create a Sleep-Conducive Environment:** Ensure your bedroom is dark, quiet, and cool to promote restful sleep.

- **Limit Screen Time Before Bed:** Exposure to blue light from screens can interfere with your ability to fall asleep. Try to avoid screens at least an hour before bed.

6. Detoxify Your Environment

Reducing exposure to environmental toxins can help prevent chronic diseases. Toxins from pesticides, plastics, pollution, and household chemicals can accumulate in the body and contribute to diseases such as cancer and autoimmune disorders. Strategies include:

- **Choose Organic Foods:** Opt for organic produce to reduce exposure to pesticides.

- **Use Natural Cleaning Products:** Switch to natural or homemade cleaning products to reduce chemical exposure in your home.

- **Filter Water and Air:** Use water and air filters to minimize exposure to pollutants and contaminants.

7. Strengthen Social Connections

Strong social connections and community support are linked to better health outcomes and longevity. Social isolation and loneliness are risk factors for chronic diseases, particularly heart disease and mental health disorders. To build strong relationships:

- **Stay Connected with Family and Friends:** Make an effort to maintain regular contact with loved ones.

- **Join Community Groups or Clubs:** Participate in activities or groups that interest you to meet like-minded people and build a sense of belonging.

- **Volunteer:** Volunteering can provide a sense of purpose and fulfillment, which contributes to overall well-being.

8. Regular Health Check-ups and Screenings

Early detection and management of risk factors like high blood pressure, high cholesterol, and prediabetes are crucial for preventing the progression of chronic diseases. Regular check-ups with your healthcare provider can help monitor your health status and catch potential issues early. Make sure to:

- **Schedule Regular Screenings:** Regular screenings for conditions like cancer, diabetes, and heart disease can help catch problems early when they are most treatable.

- **Monitor Biomarkers:** Keep track of important health metrics such as blood pressure, cholesterol levels, and blood sugar to stay informed about your health.

9. Use Herbal Remedies and Supplements Wisely

Herbal remedies and supplements can play a role in preventing and managing chronic diseases. However, they should be used with caution and under the guidance of a healthcare professional. Some beneficial options include:

- **Antioxidant Supplements:** Vitamins C and E, selenium, and other antioxidants help neutralize free radicals and reduce oxidative stress.

- **Anti-Inflammatory Herbs:** Turmeric, ginger, and green tea have anti-inflammatory properties that can help prevent chronic inflammation.

- **Probiotics:** Probiotics support gut health, which is essential for overall immunity and prevention of chronic diseases.

10. Embrace a Growth Mindset and Positive Outlook

A positive attitude and growth mindset can significantly impact your ability to prevent and reverse chronic diseases. Believing in your ability to change and improve your health encourages healthier behaviors and resilience in the face of challenges. Strategies include:

- **Practice Gratitude:** Regularly focusing on what you're grateful for can improve mental and emotional well-being.

- **Set Realistic Goals:** Break down your health goals into achievable steps to maintain motivation and avoid overwhelm.

- **Seek Support When Needed:** Don't hesitate to reach out for help from professionals, support groups, or loved ones when facing health challenges.

Preventing and reversing chronic diseases requires a multifaceted approach that addresses diet, lifestyle, environment, and mindset. By adopting these strategies, individuals can take control of their health, reduce their risk of chronic illness, and even reverse existing conditions, leading to a longer, healthier, and more vibrant life.

The Role of Lifestyle Medicine in Chronic Disease Management

Lifestyle medicine is an evidence-based approach to preventing, treating, and even reversing chronic diseases by addressing the root causes rather than merely managing symptoms. This holistic approach focuses on six key areas: nutrition, physical activity, stress management, sleep, social connections, and avoiding risky behaviors like smoking and excessive alcohol consumption. By making sustainable lifestyle changes, individuals can achieve long-term improvements in their health and well-being.

1. Nutrition as Medicine

Nutrition plays a critical role in lifestyle medicine. The emphasis is on whole, plant-based foods rich in nutrients that promote health and reduce the risk of chronic diseases such as heart disease, diabetes, and cancer. Key principles include:

- **Emphasizing Whole Foods:** Diets rich in vegetables, fruits, whole grains, nuts, seeds, and legumes provide essential vitamins, minerals, and antioxidants that help combat inflammation and oxidative stress.

- **Reducing Processed Foods and Sugars:** Processed foods and added sugars contribute to obesity, insulin resistance, and other metabolic disorders. Lifestyle medicine encourages reducing or eliminating these foods to improve overall health.

- **Personalized Nutrition Plans:** Tailoring dietary recommendations to individual needs, preferences, and medical conditions ensures that nutrition therapy is effective and sustainable.

2. Physical Activity for Prevention and Management

Regular physical activity is a cornerstone of lifestyle medicine. It helps prevent and manage a wide range of chronic conditions, including cardiovascular disease, diabetes, obesity, and mental health disorders. Key aspects include:

- **Exercise as Prescription:** Just as medications are prescribed, exercise is recommended in specific doses to address particular health concerns. For example, aerobic exercise improves cardiovascular health, while strength training helps with insulin sensitivity and bone health.

- **Incorporating Movement into Daily Life:** Encouraging patients to find enjoyable physical activities increases adherence and makes exercise a sustainable part of their lifestyle.

- **Holistic Approach to Fitness:** Integrating flexibility, balance, and strength exercises ensures a well-rounded fitness regimen that addresses all aspects of physical health.

3. Stress Management and Emotional Well-Being

Chronic stress is a significant risk factor for many diseases, including heart disease, depression, and anxiety. Lifestyle medicine emphasizes the importance of managing stress through:

- **Mindfulness and Meditation:** Techniques such as mindfulness meditation, deep breathing, and yoga help reduce stress hormones, lower blood pressure, and improve emotional resilience.

- **Cognitive Behavioral Strategies:** These strategies help individuals reframe negative thoughts and develop healthier responses to stressors.

- **Building Emotional Resilience:** Encouraging practices that enhance emotional well-being, such as gratitude journaling and fostering positive relationships, supports overall mental health.

4. Importance of Sleep

Sleep is vital for physical and mental health, yet it is often overlooked in traditional medicine. Poor sleep is linked to an increased risk of obesity, diabetes, cardiovascular disease, and impaired immune function. Lifestyle medicine addresses sleep through:

- **Sleep Hygiene Education:** Teaching patients about the importance of a regular sleep schedule, a conducive sleep environment, and minimizing screen time before bed.

- **Addressing Sleep Disorders:** Identifying and treating underlying sleep disorders, such as sleep apnea, is crucial for improving overall health outcomes.

- **Promoting Restorative Sleep:** Encouraging relaxation techniques and healthy bedtime routines to enhance sleep quality and duration.

5. Building Strong Social Connections

Social support is a powerful determinant of health. Strong relationships contribute to emotional well-being, reduce stress, and even lower the risk of chronic diseases. Lifestyle medicine encourages:

- **Strengthening Social Networks:** Encouraging patients to nurture relationships with family, friends, and community groups provides a support system that enhances overall health.

- **Community Involvement:** Participating in community activities fosters a sense of belonging and purpose, which can have positive effects on mental and physical health.

- **Combating Loneliness:** Addressing loneliness and social isolation through targeted interventions can significantly improve health outcomes.

6. Avoidance of Risky Behaviors

Lifestyle medicine also focuses on reducing or eliminating risky behaviors that contribute to chronic diseases, such as smoking, excessive alcohol consumption, and sedentary behavior. Strategies include:

- **Smoking Cessation Programs:** Providing support and resources to help individuals quit smoking is crucial for reducing the risk of respiratory and cardiovascular diseases.

- **Moderating Alcohol Intake:** Educating patients about the risks of excessive alcohol consumption and promoting moderation or abstinence as needed.

- **Encouraging Active Lifestyles:** Reducing sedentary behavior by promoting regular movement and exercise throughout the day.

7. Integrating Lifestyle Medicine into Healthcare

Lifestyle medicine is increasingly being integrated into mainstream healthcare as its benefits become more widely recognized. This involves:

- **Collaborative Care Models:** Healthcare providers, including doctors, nutritionists, exercise physiologists, and mental health professionals, work together to create comprehensive, individualized treatment plans.

- **Patient Empowerment:** Educating patients about the impact of lifestyle choices on their health empowers them to take an active role in their disease management and prevention efforts.

- **Sustainable Behavior Change:** Supporting patients in making gradual, sustainable lifestyle changes that lead to long-term health improvements.

Lifestyle medicine offers a proactive, patient-centered approach to chronic disease management that goes beyond symptom control. By focusing on the root causes of disease and promoting healthy habits, lifestyle medicine not only prevents chronic conditions but also empowers individuals to reverse existing ones, leading to a healthier, more fulfilling life.

Chapter 15: Living a Life of Vibrant Health

Cultivating Long-Term Wellness Habits

Cultivating long-term wellness habits is essential for maintaining health and preventing chronic diseases. These habits are not just about temporary fixes or quick changes; they require consistent effort and commitment to a healthy lifestyle. Here's how you can establish and sustain these habits for long-term wellness.

1. Establishing a Strong Foundation

The journey to long-term wellness begins with establishing a strong foundation of healthy habits. This involves making conscious choices that promote physical, mental, and emotional well-being.

- **Start Small and Build Gradually:** Making small, manageable changes over time is more sustainable than trying to overhaul your lifestyle all at once. For example, begin by adding one extra serving of vegetables to your daily meals or incorporating a short walk into your routine.

- **Set Realistic Goals:** Setting achievable, specific goals helps keep you motivated. Whether it's drinking more water, exercising regularly, or improving sleep, having clear goals provides direction and purpose.

- **Create a Routine:** Consistency is key to habit formation. Establishing a daily or weekly routine helps integrate wellness practices into your life, making them second nature over time.

2. Prioritizing Nutrition

Long-term wellness is heavily influenced by the foods you consume. Adopting a balanced diet rich in whole, nutrient-dense foods is crucial for maintaining energy levels, supporting immune function, and preventing disease.

- **Embrace Whole Foods:** Focus on incorporating more whole foods, such as fruits, vegetables, whole grains, lean proteins, and healthy fats, into your diet. These foods provide essential nutrients that support overall health.

- **Plan and Prepare Meals:** Meal planning and preparation can help you make healthier choices and avoid processed, convenience foods. Cooking at home allows you to control ingredients and portion sizes.

- **Mindful Eating:** Pay attention to your body's hunger and fullness cues, and savor each bite. Mindful eating helps prevent overeating and fosters a healthier relationship with food.

3. Incorporating Regular Physical Activity

Physical activity is a cornerstone of long-term wellness. It not only improves physical health but also enhances mental clarity and emotional well-being.

- **Find Activities You Enjoy:** Engaging in physical activities that you find enjoyable increases the likelihood that you will stick with them long-term. Whether it's dancing, hiking, swimming, or yoga, choose activities that bring you joy.

- **Mix It Up:** Variety in your exercise routine prevents boredom and helps you work different muscle groups. Combine cardio, strength training, flexibility exercises, and balance activities for a well-rounded fitness program.

- **Make Movement a Habit:** Incorporate movement into your daily life by taking the stairs, walking or biking instead of driving short distances, or doing a quick stretch break during work hours.

4. Managing Stress Effectively

Chronic stress can have detrimental effects on your health, making stress management an essential component of long-term wellness.

- **Practice Relaxation Techniques:** Techniques such as deep breathing, meditation, progressive muscle relaxation, and guided imagery can help reduce stress and promote relaxation.

- **Prioritize Downtime:** Make time for activities that help you unwind, whether it's reading a book, spending time in nature, or engaging in a hobby. Regular downtime is crucial for mental and emotional recovery.

- **Build Emotional Resilience:** Developing resilience through positive thinking, gratitude practices, and cultivating strong social connections helps you navigate life's challenges more effectively.

5. Ensuring Adequate Sleep

Quality sleep is fundamental to long-term health. It's during sleep that your body repairs itself, consolidates memories, and regulates hormones.

- **Establish a Sleep Routine:** Going to bed and waking up at the same time each day, even on weekends, helps regulate your body's internal clock and improve sleep quality.

- **Create a Sleep-Conducive Environment:** Ensure your bedroom is quiet, dark, and cool. Invest in a comfortable mattress and pillows, and remove distractions such as electronic devices.

- **Address Sleep Issues:** If you struggle with sleep, it's important to address underlying issues such as insomnia, sleep apnea, or restless leg syndrome. Seeking help from a healthcare professional can improve your sleep quality and overall health.

6. Fostering Positive Relationships

Social connections are a vital aspect of long-term wellness. Strong relationships provide emotional support, reduce stress, and contribute to a sense of belonging.

- **Nurture Your Relationships:** Invest time and effort into building and maintaining relationships with family, friends, and community members. Meaningful connections are essential for emotional well-being.

- **Communicate Openly:** Effective communication is key to healthy relationships. Practice active listening, express your thoughts and feelings clearly, and resolve conflicts in a constructive manner.

- **Seek Support:** Don't hesitate to seek support when you need it. Whether it's confiding in a friend, joining a support group, or seeking professional counseling, reaching out is a sign of strength.

7. Embracing Lifelong Learning

Adopting a mindset of lifelong learning can enhance your overall well-being by keeping your mind active and engaged.

- **Stay Curious:** Continuously seek out new knowledge and experiences. Whether it's learning a new skill, exploring a hobby, or staying informed about health and wellness trends, staying curious promotes mental agility and growth.

- **Adapt and Evolve:** Be open to change and adapt your wellness habits as needed. As you move through different stages of life, your needs and priorities may shift, requiring adjustments to your routine.

- **Celebrate Progress:** Acknowledge and celebrate your achievements, no matter how small. Recognizing your progress reinforces positive behavior and keeps you motivated to continue on your wellness journey.

Cultivating long-term wellness habits is a continuous process that requires dedication and self-awareness. By establishing a strong foundation, prioritizing nutrition, incorporating regular physical activity, managing stress, ensuring adequate sleep, fostering positive relationships, and embracing lifelong learning, you can create a sustainable and fulfilling lifestyle. These habits not only enhance your current well-being but also contribute to your overall health and longevity.

Finding Joy and Purpose in Healthful Living

Living a healthful life is about more than just following a routine of nutritious eating, regular exercise, and good sleep. It's about finding joy and purpose in the choices you make every day. When healthful living is infused with positivity and meaning, it becomes a source of happiness and fulfillment rather than a series of obligations. Here's how you can cultivate joy and purpose in your wellness journey.

1. Aligning Wellness with Personal Values

The first step in finding joy and purpose in healthful living is to align your wellness practices with your personal values and beliefs.

- **Identify Your Core Values:** Reflect on what matters most to you. Whether it's family, community, environmental sustainability, or spiritual growth, understanding your core values helps you make healthful living more meaningful.

- **Make Choices That Reflect Your Values:** Once you've identified your values, align your daily habits with them. For example, if you value sustainability, you might choose to eat locally-sourced, organic foods or reduce waste by opting for reusable products.

- **Embrace Authenticity:** Living authentically, in a way that feels true to who you are, brings a sense of purpose and joy. Let go of societal expectations or trends that don't resonate with you and focus on what genuinely makes you feel good.

2. Finding Joy in Daily Healthful Practices

Healthful living doesn't have to be a chore; it can be a joyful and rewarding experience.

- **Create Enjoyable Routines:** Incorporate activities into your routine that you genuinely enjoy. Whether it's a morning yoga session, cooking a delicious meal, or taking a nature walk, make time for practices that bring you happiness.

- **Savor the Moment:** Practice mindfulness in your daily activities. By being fully present and engaged in what you're doing, whether it's eating a meal or working out, you can find greater satisfaction and joy in the moment.

- **Celebrate Small Wins:** Recognize and celebrate your achievements, no matter how small. Whether you've made a healthy meal, completed a workout, or simply taken time to relax, acknowledging these efforts boosts your motivation and joy.

3. Connecting Healthful Living with a Larger Purpose

Healthful living becomes more meaningful when it's connected to a larger purpose or goal.

- **Contribute to a Greater Cause:** Consider how your healthful practices can contribute to the well-being of others or the planet. For instance, growing your own food not only nourishes you but also reduces your environmental footprint.

- **Set Meaningful Goals:** Set goals that extend beyond physical health, such as building stronger relationships, contributing to your community, or pursuing a passion. Achieving these goals can bring a deeper sense of fulfillment and purpose.

- **Inspire and Educate Others:** Share your healthful living journey with others. By inspiring friends, family, or even a wider community to adopt healthier habits, you contribute to a ripple effect of positive change.

4. Cultivating Gratitude and Positivity

Gratitude and positivity are powerful tools for finding joy in healthful living.

- **Practice Gratitude Daily:** Take time each day to reflect on what you're grateful for. This can be as simple as appreciating the taste of a healthy meal, the beauty of nature, or the support of loved ones. Gratitude shifts your focus to the positive aspects of your life, enhancing your overall sense of well-being.

- **Reframe Challenges as Opportunities:** Rather than viewing health challenges as setbacks, see them as opportunities for growth and learning. Adopting a positive mindset can help you navigate difficulties with resilience and grace.

- **Surround Yourself with Positivity:** Engage with people, activities, and environments that uplift you. Positive influences reinforce your commitment to healthful living and make the journey more enjoyable.

5. Integrating Joy and Purpose into Your Community

Healthful living is not just an individual pursuit; it's also about connecting with others and building a supportive community.

- **Share Joyful Experiences:** Engage in activities that promote health and well-being with others. Whether it's a group fitness class, a cooking workshop, or a community garden, sharing these experiences fosters a sense of connection and joy.

- **Support Others on Their Journey:** Offer encouragement and support to those around you who are also striving to live healthfully. Being part of a supportive network not only enhances your own well-being but also brings a sense of purpose and fulfillment.

- **Celebrate Together:** Celebrate milestones and successes with your community. Whether it's completing a fitness challenge, reaching a personal health goal, or simply enjoying a healthy meal together, shared celebrations amplify the joy of healthful living.

Finding joy and purpose in healthful living is about more than just following a set of guidelines; it's about creating a lifestyle that is deeply fulfilling and aligned with your values. By integrating joy into your daily practices, connecting with a larger purpose, cultivating gratitude and positivity, and engaging with your community, you can transform healthful living into a rich and rewarding journey. This approach not only enhances your well-being but also brings lasting happiness and meaning to your life.

Inspiring Stories of Transformation

Stories of transformation are powerful reminders that change is possible, no matter how difficult the journey may seem. They inspire us to believe in our potential and remind us that we are capable of overcoming obstacles to achieve our goals. These stories offer a glimpse into the lives of individuals who have embraced healthful living, made significant changes, and found joy and fulfillment along the way.

1. Overcoming Chronic Illness

Sarah's story is one of resilience and determination. For years, she struggled with chronic fatigue syndrome and irritable bowel syndrome (IBS). These conditions left her feeling exhausted and in constant discomfort, with little hope for a better future. After countless visits to doctors and specialists, Sarah decided to take control of her health through lifestyle changes.

- **The Shift:** Sarah began by researching holistic health practices and discovered the importance of nutrition, stress management, and detoxification. She eliminated processed foods, refined sugars, and gluten from her diet, replacing them with whole, organic foods. She also incorporated regular exercise and began practicing mindfulness and meditation to manage stress.

- **The Transformation:** Over time, Sarah's symptoms began to diminish. Her energy levels increased, and her digestive issues improved significantly. By embracing a holistic approach to health, she not only managed her conditions but also regained control of her life. Today, Sarah is an advocate for holistic health and shares her journey to inspire others.

2. Reversing Type 2 Diabetes

John's journey is a testament to the power of diet and lifestyle in managing chronic conditions. Diagnosed with type 2 diabetes at the age of 45, John was told he would need to rely on medication for the rest of his life. Determined to avoid this path, he decided to explore alternative options.

- **The Shift:** John began by adopting a low-carbohydrate, high-fat (LCHF) diet, which focused on whole, unprocessed foods. He eliminated sugars, refined grains, and starchy vegetables, and started incorporating more healthy fats, lean proteins, and non-starchy vegetables into his meals. In addition to dietary changes, John committed to daily exercise and began practicing intermittent fasting.

- **The Transformation:** Within months, John experienced dramatic improvements in his blood sugar levels, allowing him to reduce his reliance on medication. Over time, his doctor confirmed that he had reversed his diabetes through lifestyle changes. John's success has inspired many others in his community to explore dietary approaches to managing and even reversing chronic conditions.

3. Healing Through Mindset and Spiritual Growth

Maria's story highlights the profound impact of mindset and spiritual health on physical well-being. After a traumatic loss, Maria found herself in a deep depression, which manifested in physical ailments such as chronic pain and fatigue. Traditional treatments offered little relief, prompting her to explore alternative healing methods.

- **The Shift:** Maria began attending a spiritual retreat where she learned about the power of positive thinking, gratitude, and self-compassion. She started practicing daily affirmations, meditation, and journaling to process her emotions and shift her mindset. She also sought out therapy and engaged in community support groups.

- **The Transformation:** As Maria's mindset shifted, so did her physical health. Her pain and fatigue gradually diminished, and she began to feel more energetic and hopeful. By focusing on her mental and spiritual health, Maria was able to transform her life and find peace and joy again. Her journey serves as a reminder of the interconnectedness of mind, body, and spirit in the healing process.

4. Reclaiming Health After a Life of Stress and Poor Habits

Tom had spent most of his adult life working in a high-stress corporate environment, where long hours and poor dietary choices were the norm. By the time he reached his mid-50s, he was overweight, hypertensive, and at risk for heart disease. Realizing that he needed to make drastic changes, Tom decided to prioritize his health.

- **The Shift:** Tom began by enrolling in a wellness program that focused on balanced nutrition, regular exercise, and stress management techniques. He replaced his fast-food meals with home-cooked, nutrient-dense dishes, started walking every morning, and learned techniques like deep breathing and yoga to manage stress.

- **The Transformation:** Within a year, Tom lost a significant amount of weight, lowered his blood pressure, and reduced his risk for heart disease. He felt more energetic and balanced, both physically and mentally. Tom's story is an inspiring example of how it's never too late to make meaningful changes and reclaim one's health.

5. Embracing a Holistic Lifestyle for Long-Term Wellness

Linda's transformation is a testament to the power of holistic living. After years of struggling with anxiety, insomnia, and digestive issues, Linda decided to take a comprehensive approach to her health.

- **The Shift:** Linda began by overhauling her diet, focusing on organic, whole foods, and eliminating processed foods, caffeine, and alcohol. She incorporated regular exercise, such as yoga and walking, into her routine. Additionally, Linda practiced mindfulness meditation and sought support from a holistic health coach to guide her journey.

- **The Transformation:** Over time, Linda's anxiety diminished, her sleep improved, and her digestive issues resolved. She discovered a sense of peace and balance that had been missing from her life for years. By embracing a holistic lifestyle, Linda not only improved her physical health but also found greater emotional and spiritual well-being.

These inspiring stories of transformation demonstrate that with determination, the right mindset, and a holistic approach, it is possible to overcome significant health challenges and live a vibrant, fulfilling life. Each journey is unique, but the common thread is the commitment to embracing healthful living in all its facets. These stories remind us that change is possible, and they encourage us to take the first step toward our own transformations.

Conclusion: Your Journey to Optimal Health

Reflecting on the SUSTAIN ME Principles

As you reach the conclusion of this journey through the SUSTAIN ME principles, it's important to take a moment to reflect on what you've learned and how these principles can be integrated into your life. The SUSTAIN ME approach is not just a set of guidelines; it's a comprehensive philosophy of wellness that embraces every aspect of your being, from the physical to the mental and emotional.

1. The Holistic Nature of SUSTAIN ME

The SUSTAIN ME principles are designed to work together, creating a holistic approach to health and well-being. Each principle—Sustenance, Unwind, Sleep, Toxin Elimination, Activity, Immune Support, Nourish, Mindset, and Empower—addresses a different aspect of your health, but they are all interconnected. By reflecting on how these principles interrelate, you can see how changes in one area can positively influence others. For example:

- **Nutrition (Sustenance)** affects your energy levels, immune function, and even your mood, demonstrating the connection between diet and overall well-being.

- **Stress Management (Unwind)** is crucial for mental clarity and emotional stability, which in turn supports physical health by reducing inflammation and improving sleep quality.

- **Mindset and Empowerment** are essential for sustaining long-term health changes, helping you to stay motivated and resilient in the face of challenges.

Understanding the synergy between these principles helps you create a more balanced and sustainable approach to health.

2. The Personalization of Wellness

One of the core tenets of SUSTAIN ME is that wellness is personal. The principles provide a framework, but how you apply them will depend on your unique needs, goals, and circumstances. Reflecting on your journey, consider:

- **Which principles resonated most with you?** Perhaps you found particular value in the dietary guidance, or maybe the emphasis on mindfulness and stress management was most impactful.

- **What changes have you noticed in your health and well-being?** Take stock of how your body and mind have responded to the integration of these principles. Are you feeling more energized, less stressed, or more in control of your health?

- **How have your priorities shifted?** As you've learned more about the holistic approach to wellness, you may find that your goals and priorities have evolved. Reflect on what matters most to you now and how the SUSTAIN ME principles align with those values.

By personalizing the principles to fit your life, you create a wellness plan that is both effective and sustainable.

3. The Journey of Continuous Growth

Wellness is not a destination but a journey of continuous growth and improvement. The SUSTAIN ME principles are tools that you can use throughout your life, adapting them as your needs change. Reflect on:

- **The progress you've made so far.** Celebrate the small victories and the positive changes you've implemented. Whether you've improved your diet, reduced stress, or adopted a more positive mindset, these steps are important milestones on your wellness journey.

- **The challenges you've faced.** Reflect on the obstacles that have come up along the way and how you've addressed them. What have you learned from these challenges, and how can you use that knowledge moving forward?

- **The future of your wellness journey.** Consider how you will continue to apply the SUSTAIN ME principles in the future. What areas would you like to focus on next? How can you keep growing and evolving in your pursuit of optimal health?

By viewing wellness as an ongoing process, you stay open to learning, adapting, and growing.

4. The Importance of Community and Support

Reflecting on your journey, recognize the importance of community and support in sustaining healthful living. Whether it's family, friends, or a broader community, having a support system can make a significant difference in your ability to maintain positive changes.

- **Who has supported you on this journey?** Reflect on the people who have encouraged and motivated you. How can you continue to nurture these relationships?

- **How can you support others?** Consider how you can share what you've learned with others, inspiring them to embark on their own wellness journeys. Whether it's through sharing recipes, offering encouragement, or simply being a role model, you have the power to positively influence those around you.

A strong support system helps you stay accountable and motivated, making it easier to sustain healthful habits over the long term.

5. Embracing the SUSTAIN ME Lifestyle

Finally, reflecting on the SUSTAIN ME principles is about embracing this lifestyle as a way of life, not just a temporary change. This holistic approach to wellness is designed to be sustainable, helping you achieve and maintain optimal health over the long term.

- **Commitment to lifelong wellness.** Embrace the idea that healthful living is a lifelong journey. By committing to the SUSTAIN ME principles, you are investing in your long-term health and well-being.

- **Flexibility and adaptation.** Recognize that life is dynamic, and your wellness plan should be flexible enough to adapt to changes in your life. The SUSTAIN ME principles provide a foundation, but it's up to you to adapt them as your needs evolve.

- **Living with intention.** Reflect on the importance of living with intention, making conscious choices that align with your values and health goals. By embracing the SUSTAIN ME lifestyle, you are choosing to prioritize your health and well-being, creating a life that is both fulfilling and sustainable.

Reflecting on the SUSTAIN ME principles is an opportunity to appreciate the progress you've made, understand the interconnectedness of these principles, and recommit to your wellness journey. This holistic approach to health is not just about avoiding illness, but about thriving in all aspects of your life—physically, mentally, and emotionally. By continuing to apply and adapt these principles, you are taking proactive steps toward a healthier, happier, and more balanced life.

Continuing Your Wellness Journey

Embarking on a wellness journey is just the beginning; the real work lies in maintaining and evolving your health practices over time. The principles of SUSTAIN ME provide a solid foundation, but ongoing commitment and adaptability are key to achieving and sustaining long-term well-being. Here's how you can continue your wellness journey effectively:

1. Setting Long-Term Health Goals

To ensure continued progress, it's essential to set and regularly revisit long-term health goals. These goals should be realistic, measurable, and aligned with your personal values and aspirations.

- **Define Clear Objectives:** Outline specific health goals that you want to achieve in the coming months or years. For instance, you might aim to maintain a balanced diet, consistently exercise, or enhance mental well-being.

- **Break Down Goals into Actionable Steps:** Divide your long-term goals into smaller, manageable tasks. For example, if your goal is to improve your physical fitness, you might start with a goal of exercising three times a week and gradually increase as you progress.

- **Review and Adjust:** Regularly assess your progress towards your goals. Celebrate milestones and make adjustments as needed based on your experiences and any changes in your circumstances.

2. Adapting to Life's Changes

Life is dynamic, and so should be your approach to wellness. Adapting your wellness plan to fit different stages of life and varying circumstances is crucial for sustained success.

- **Recognize Life Transitions:** Major life events, such as changing jobs, moving to a new place, or experiencing personal milestones, can impact your wellness routine. Acknowledge these transitions and adjust your plan accordingly.

- **Stay Flexible:** Allow room for flexibility in your wellness plan. Life's unpredictability means that you might need to modify your routines and goals as you navigate new challenges or opportunities.

- **Prioritize Self-Compassion:** Be kind to yourself during times of change. Understand that it's okay to face setbacks and that progress is not always linear. Embrace a compassionate approach towards yourself as you adapt.

3. Expanding Your Knowledge and Practices

Continuing your wellness journey involves a commitment to ongoing learning and growth. Expand your knowledge and practices to enrich your health and well-being.

- **Stay Informed:** Keep up-to-date with the latest research and trends in health and wellness. Read books, attend workshops, and follow credible sources that provide new insights and evidence-based practices.

- **Explore New Techniques:** Experiment with new wellness techniques or practices that align with your interests and needs. This could include trying different types of exercise, exploring new mindfulness practices, or integrating new nutritional approaches.

- **Seek Professional Guidance:** Consult with health professionals, such as dietitians, fitness trainers, or therapists, to gain expert advice tailored to your specific needs. They can provide valuable support and help you refine your wellness plan.

4. Building and Nurturing Support Networks

A strong support network can significantly enhance your wellness journey. Surround yourself with individuals and communities that encourage and support your efforts.

- **Connect with Like-Minded Individuals:** Engage with communities or groups that share your health goals and values. This could include joining fitness clubs, online forums, or local wellness groups.

- **Seek Accountability Partners:** Find friends or family members who can support you and hold you accountable to your goals. Regular check-ins and shared activities can keep you motivated and committed.

- **Offer Support to Others:** Share your journey and insights with others who may be on their own wellness paths. By supporting and encouraging others, you can reinforce your own commitment and contribute to a positive community environment.

5. Embracing a Holistic Approach

Continuing your wellness journey means maintaining a holistic approach to health. Integrate all aspects of the SUSTAIN ME principles into your daily life to create a balanced and sustainable lifestyle.

- **Integrate Wellness into Daily Life:** Make wellness a natural part of your routine by incorporating healthy habits into your daily activities. This might include meal planning, regular exercise, and mindfulness practices.

- **Cultivate Balance:** Strive for balance in all areas of your life, including work, relationships, and personal interests. A balanced life supports overall well-being and prevents burnout.

- **Foster a Positive Mindset:** Keep a positive and proactive mindset towards your health journey. Embrace challenges as opportunities for growth and maintain an optimistic outlook on your progress.

6. Reflecting and Celebrating Your Journey

Regular reflection and celebration of your achievements are essential for maintaining motivation and acknowledging the progress you've made.

- **Journal Your Progress:** Keep a journal to document your experiences, challenges, and successes. Reflecting on your journey can provide valuable insights and reinforce your commitment to your goals.

- **Celebrate Milestones:** Recognize and celebrate your achievements, no matter how small. Celebrating milestones can boost your motivation and remind you of the positive impact of your efforts.

- **Practice Gratitude:** Cultivate a sense of gratitude for the positive changes in your life. Appreciating your progress and the support you've received can enhance your overall sense of well-being.

Continuing your wellness journey involves a dynamic interplay of setting goals, adapting to changes, expanding your knowledge, building support networks, embracing a holistic approach, and reflecting on your progress. By integrating these practices into your daily life, you can sustain your commitment to health and well-being, creating a fulfilling and balanced lifestyle. Remember that wellness is a lifelong journey, and every step you take contributes to a healthier, happier you.

Encouraging Others to Embrace a Holistic Lifestyle

Sharing the principles of holistic wellness and inspiring others to embrace a balanced, health-focused lifestyle can be profoundly rewarding. Your enthusiasm and commitment to a holistic approach can positively influence those around you, leading them to explore and integrate these practices into their own lives. Here's how you can effectively encourage others to adopt a holistic lifestyle:

1. Lead by Example

One of the most powerful ways to inspire others is by demonstrating the benefits of a holistic lifestyle through your own actions.

- **Showcase Your Journey:** Share your personal experiences and successes with friends, family, or colleagues. Highlight how adopting holistic practices has improved your overall well-being.

- **Practice What You Preach:** Consistently incorporate the SUSTAIN ME principles into your daily life. Your visible commitment to healthful living can serve as a compelling example for others.

- **Share Positive Outcomes:** Discuss the positive changes you've experienced, such as increased energy, better mood, or improved health markers. Concrete examples of how holistic practices have benefited you can motivate others to give them a try.

2. Educate and Inform

Providing information and education about the benefits of a holistic lifestyle can help others understand and appreciate the value of these practices.

- **Organize Workshops and Seminars:** Host workshops or seminars on topics related to holistic health, such as nutrition, stress management, or mindfulness. These events can provide valuable information and practical tips to participants.

- **Create Informative Content:** Share articles, blogs, or social media posts that highlight the principles of holistic wellness. Include practical advice, success stories, and research findings to engage and educate your audience.

- **Recommend Resources:** Suggest books, podcasts, or online courses that cover holistic health topics. Offering a range of resources allows individuals to explore areas of interest at their own pace.

3. Foster a Supportive Community

Building a community that values holistic health can create a supportive environment for others to explore and adopt these practices.

- **Form Support Groups:** Establish support groups or wellness communities where individuals can share experiences, seek advice, and offer encouragement. These groups can provide a sense of belonging and accountability.

- **Encourage Group Activities:** Organize group activities such as fitness classes, cooking demonstrations, or meditation sessions. Group activities can make holistic practices more accessible and enjoyable.

- **Promote Shared Goals:** Encourage friends and family to set and pursue shared wellness goals. Working together towards common objectives can strengthen motivation and create a sense of camaraderie.

4. Offer Practical Tips and Support

Providing practical guidance and support can make it easier for others to incorporate holistic practices into their lives.

- **Share Simple Strategies:** Offer easy-to-implement tips for integrating holistic practices, such as meal planning, stress reduction techniques, or sleep improvement strategies. Simplicity can help overcome initial barriers to change.

- **Provide Personalized Advice:** Tailor your recommendations to individual needs and preferences. Personalized advice can address specific challenges and make holistic practices more relevant and manageable.

- **Be Available for Guidance:** Offer to answer questions, provide feedback, and support those who are exploring holistic practices. Your availability and encouragement can make a significant difference in their journey.

5. Celebrate Progress and Success

Recognizing and celebrating progress can boost motivation and reinforce positive behavior.

- **Acknowledge Milestones:** Celebrate achievements, both big and small, to encourage continued efforts. Acknowledging progress can provide a sense of accomplishment and motivation to keep going.

- **Share Success Stories:** Highlight stories of individuals who have successfully adopted a holistic lifestyle. Success stories can inspire and validate the benefits of holistic practices.

- **Encourage Reflection:** Invite others to reflect on their own progress and the positive changes they've experienced. Reflection can help solidify their commitment to holistic health.

6. Address Misconceptions and Challenges

Be prepared to address common misconceptions and challenges related to holistic health.

- **Provide Evidence-Based Information:** Address misconceptions with accurate, evidence-based information. Clarify any misunderstandings and provide reliable sources to support your explanations.

- **Offer Solutions to Challenges:** Help others overcome obstacles they may face in adopting a holistic lifestyle. Whether it's finding time for exercise or navigating dietary changes, offer practical solutions and support.

- **Promote a Balanced Approach:** Emphasize that holistic health is about balance and gradual change, not perfection. Encourage a flexible and realistic approach to integrating new practices into daily life.

Encouraging others to embrace a holistic lifestyle involves leading by example, educating and informing, fostering community, offering practical support, celebrating progress, and addressing challenges. By sharing your passion for holistic health and providing practical guidance, you can inspire and support others in their own wellness journeys. Embracing a holistic approach is not just about improving individual well-being; it's about creating a ripple effect that positively impacts the health and happiness of those around you.

Made in the USA
Middletown, DE
03 September 2024

59931590R00117